the THIRLBY

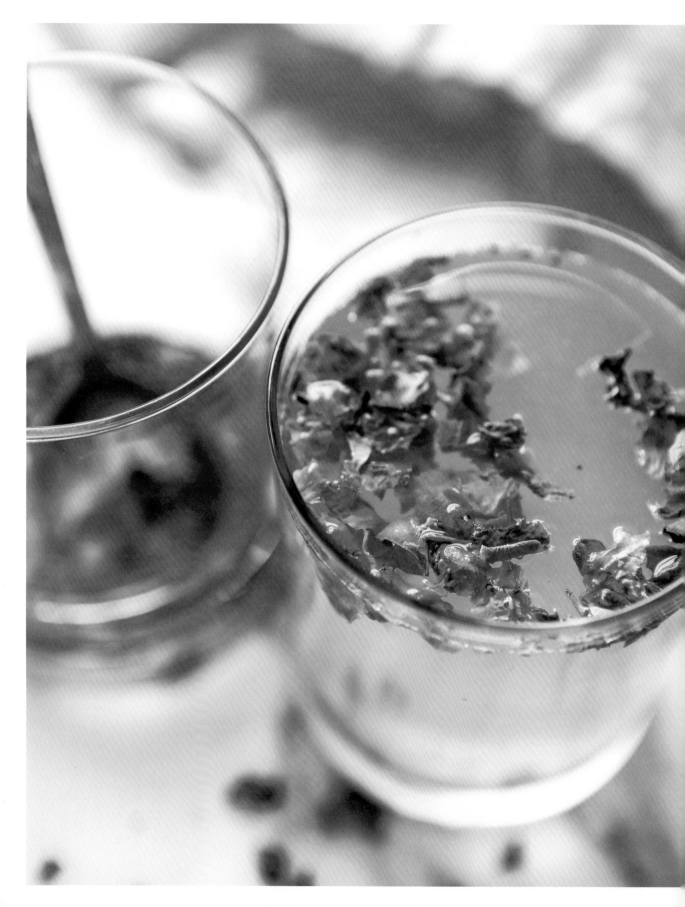

the

THIRLBY

A FIELD GUIDE TO A VIBRANT MIND, BODY, & SOUL

ALMILA KAKINC-DODD

PRESTEL

MUNICH LONDON NEW YORK

© Prestel Verlag, Munich · London · New York 2018
A member of Verlagsgruppe Random House GmbH
Neumarkter Strasse 28 · 81673 Munich

Prestel Publishing Ltd.
14-17 Wells Street
London W1T 3PD

Prestel Publishing
900 Broadway, Suite 603
New York, NY 10003

Library of Congress Cataloging-in-Publication Data

Names: Kakinc-Dodd, Almila, author.
Title: The Thirlby : a field guide to a vibrant mind, body, and soul / Almila
Kakinc-Dodd.
Description: Munich ; New York : Prestel, [2018] | Includes bibliographical
references and index.
Identifiers: LCCN 2017032795 | ISBN 9783791383910 (hardcover)
Subjects: LCSH: Health. | Beauty, Personal. | Mind and body. | Well-being.
Classification: LCC RA776 .K2125 2017 | DDC 613--dc23
LC record available at https://lccn.loc.gov/2017032795

A CIP catalogue record for this book is available from the British Library.

Editorial direction: Holly La Due
Cover and interior design: Laura Palese
Production management: Luke Chase
Copyediting: John Son, Lauren Salkeld
Proofreading: Monica Parcell
Index: Marilyn Bliss

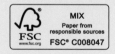

Verlagsgruppe Random House FSC® N001967

Printed in China

ISBN: 978-3-7913-8391-0

www.prestel.com

To my mother,

who cleared paths full of thorns so that
her daughters may flower.

Thank you, Mama, for showing me
how to feel love, be love, and see love—not only
for others but most importantly, for myself.

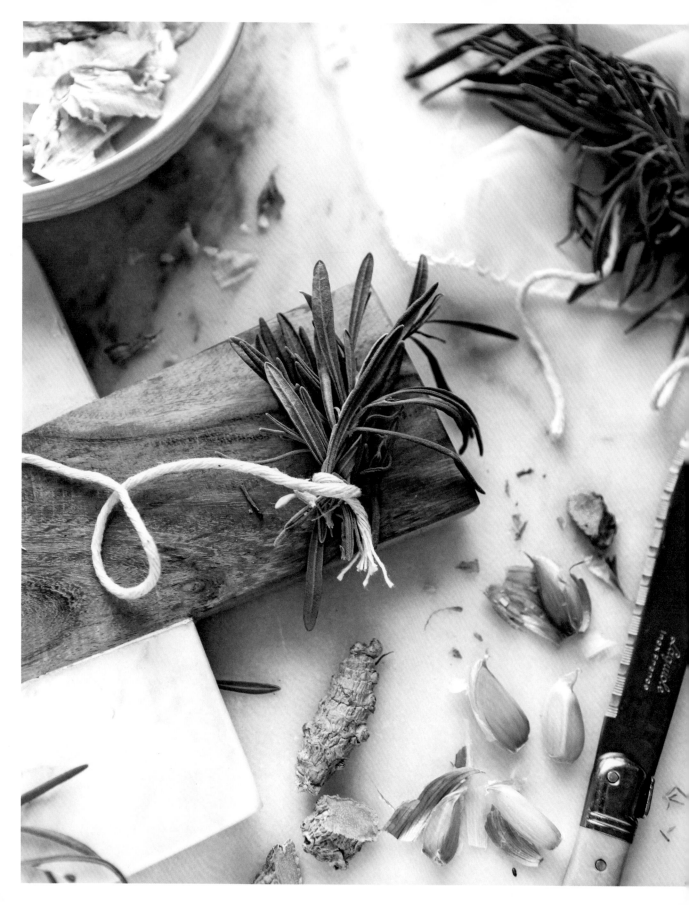

CONTENTS

INTRODUCTION

People often ask me

THE MEANING OF THIRLBY.

There is no definition, it's simply a name. I chose it in my initial venture into blogging on style at the unripe age of fourteen. I love *Thirlby* precisely because it is not tied down by a specific definition. It's a name that exists simply as a gathering of letters that I find whimsical, beautiful, and tuneful. It sounds like twirling—and who doesn't love the delight of that? So, *Thirlby* was and still is a curation of all that I find aesthetically pleasing, all that is beautiful in its sheer and undefinable state. That is what I try to cultivate within my life and hope to do so in yours with this book: to find beauty and live within it without having to define or explain it in any way. Simply absorbing, being, and appreciating the moment. May this book rushing out of my heart expand yours—*that is my mission.*

Transplanted from the straits of the Bosphorus to the brick-and-mortar of Georgetown, Washington, DC, on a night's notice at the age of ten, my life quickly resembled Istanbul's Eurasian divide. Afloat at the crossroads of two disparate cultures, I cultivated a home in my heart. There I could unfurl my vision. Missing the Matisse prints of our home in Istanbul, I enrolled in painting and art classes.

I found that in sculpting bodies with my brush I could escape the travails of mine.

It seemed my body was afflicted with not only the traumas of puberty and geographical dislocation, but with an illness that further disconnected my presence from the liminal, stateless space it occupied. My body felt like an unwelcome weight, and I tried to control it by developing anorexia. Later, during a second bout of anorexia, I was diagnosed with celiac disease, an autoimmune condition that not only robbed me of my ability to consume gluten, but also any remaining connection I had to my body. Not only was my body deprived of food by my own volition, but now I had a host of allergies. I couldn't eat dairy, gluten, grains, soy, legumes, nightshades, or coffee.

As I became physically and metaphorically thinner, my body's significance was reduced to a mere abstraction. My body had been separated from the self into things that can be technically calculated, organized, and planned—optimal numbers on a scale, waistline measurements, calories. Adhering to these ideals required great willpower. My mind became a tool to hack into an unruly

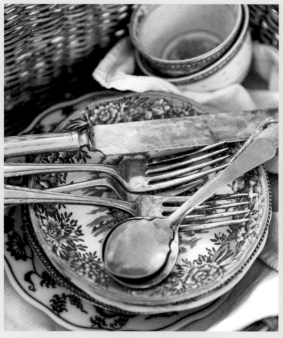 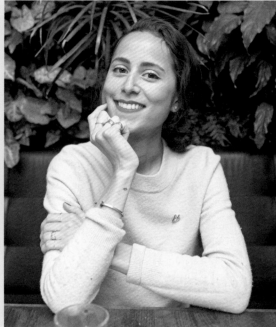

body, an entity whose structure could not be solved. It was an attempt to locate control paradoxically through disorder and disease.

My ideal self lived in the healing body of the present. My disordered self desired to consume me into the past. My unrealized future self morphed into a ghostly figure in between.

Asking what a body is became untenable to me. Such questions were based on the assumption that the body was a "substance" that could be known and defined. I came to realize that disease cannot be managed through calculated control of the body. This is because the body is multiple; it is not tissues, blood and bones, mind over body, hunger over stomach pangs, parts to be enacted, or symptoms to manage. Rather, the body is always in movement and in dynamic

process. There are experiences of the body that suggest that there may be immateriality that cannot be articulated. The body is "open, relational, human and non-human, material and immaterial, sentient, and processual," says Lisa Blackman in her book *The Body*. It is undefinable—*Thirlby*.

This guidebook honors the ways in which we attempt to hang together a coherent sense of self in the face of multiplicity. To find both timelessness in traditional recipes and a second-slice delight in the measured labor of a cake. To wear equally the perfumed red blouse on a hanger and a T-shirt on the back of a chair—the musky fibers of worn days. To bottle tinctures and kombucha and oils but uncork emotions. In a life governed by measurements—of our body, our blood, our food—let this book be a solace to lead you into a life unmeasured.

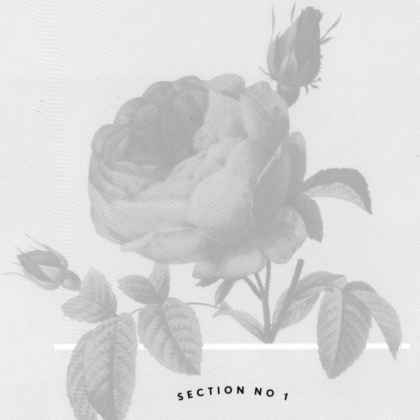

SECTION NO 1

FARMACY

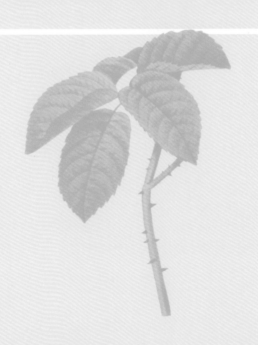

IN THE SURGE *of our* DAILY LIVES,

we often stay afloat with the paddles of convenience, habit, or ignorance. When facing illness or discomfort, we unthinkingly reach toward an over-the-counter painkiller. In the pained itch of a breakout, we might scratch for the acne remedies of our pubescent past.

This section is a hand of compassion to lead us out of habits that may be doing a disservice to our bodies, whether it's the toxic chemicals in our household products or the toxic thoughts that we house within ourselves. My intention is to guide you toward alternative modalities that will address your needs holistically.

It's a section to reconnect life to the body that lives it, to cycle back to ourselves and to return to a time when the farm was our pharmacy, where we drew our medicine from food, plants, and our planet. Yet, it's a mindful approach. The time we live in is not then but now, where medical technology can eradicate disease and treat innumerable disorders. This section is a guide meant to complement our health care, not replace it whole cloth, or to take a dogmatic and static approach to it. May it be a resource to gather the wisdom of the past in the present to revive your future.

You will notice that throughout the book my recommendations and claims include footnotes. This is my commitment to provide credible research and point you towards continued study if you're interested. Scientific literature on holistic health is growing rapidly and I encourage you to explore it.

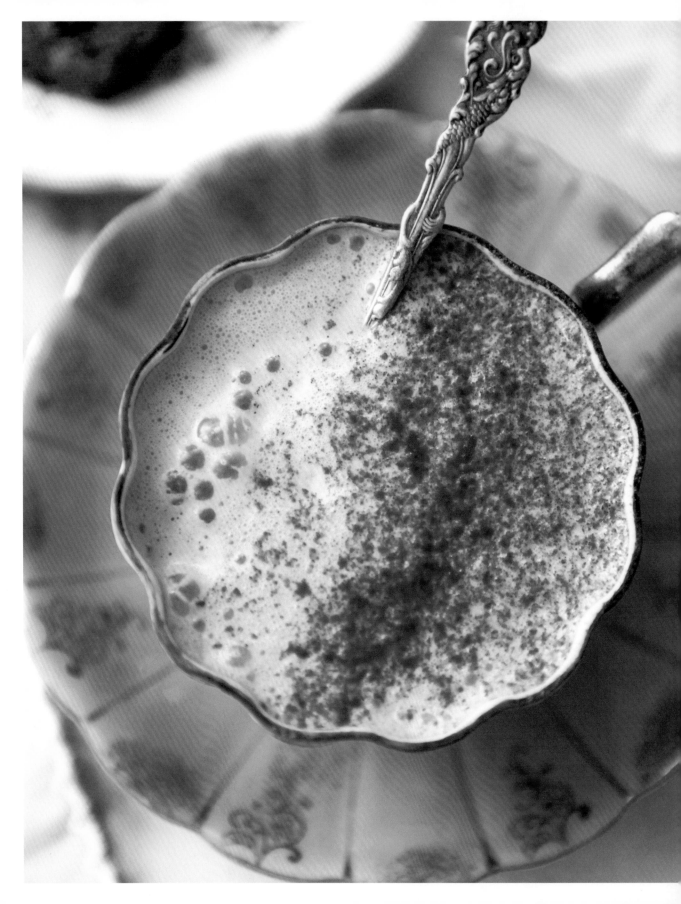

AUTOIMMUNE PROTOCOL

When I was diagnosed with celiac disease, I was already physiologically and emotionally depleted. Most autoimmune conditions wage a silent self-inflicted attack on the tissues, such as those in the gut, because the body is no longer able to differentiate the good guys from the bad guys. This can go on for a while before any symptoms of the disease occur.

In my case, I received my diagnosis in the throes of a body already damaged from anorexia. Not only had my body been malnourished but the nutrition it did receive was not being absorbed. Removing gluten didn't help because I continued to eat other foods that inflamed a hypersensitive and compromised digestive system.[1] Elimination diets did not help either because they do not address all the immune triggers in a gut inflamed by autoimmune disease.[2]

What brought me into healing was the **AUTOIMMUNE PROTOCOL (AIP) DIET**, which directly focuses on restoring intestinal mucosa and reducing inflammation. Although it's not a cure—as there is none for autoimmune conditions—AIP can help bring about remission.

A word of caution: nutrition alone will not address autoimmune symptoms. Supplements that support proper adrenal and insulin function (which are often compromised), reducing stress levels, and working with a skilled practitioner can be part of one's overall approach to managing an autoimmune condition.

The autoimmune protocol is intricately outlined in Dr. Sarah Ballantyne's *The Paleo Approach*. In short, it consists of multiple phases, which include eliminating certain foods that irritate the gut and aggravate an already dysbiotic gut. Removing these triggers also addresses the **GUT ASSOCIATED LYMPHOID TISSUE (GALT)**. The intestines contain 70 percent of these tissues that moderate immune response by producing antigens or antibodies, like those against gluten. The elimination of trigger foods reduces this reactionary GALT process from occurring, thereby calming both the digestive and immune system. Below is a basic list of foods to eliminate from Phase One of the AIP diet. Once you see results, you can move on to Phases Two and Three in *The Paleo Approach*.

Nuts and seeds (including their oils and spices such as cacao, cumin, mustard, and coriander)

Legumes (including soy)

Grains (including gluten-free ones)

Alternative sweeteners (including stevia, xylitol, erythritol, and maple syrup)

Dried fruits with a limit of two per day of fresh fruits

Dairy products and eggs

Alcohol

Nightshades, including tomato, potato (but not sweet potato), eggplant, hot peppers, goji berries, ashwagandha, and more

DIGESTION & GUT-FRIENDLY STAPLES

By the time I received my celiac diagnosis, my digestive tract was a wreck. The lining of my small intestine had been damaged by my immune system reacting to the gluten protein, atrophying the intestinal villi that aid assimilation. My digestion was slow, and consequently I felt slow, too.

If you regularly experience diarrhea, constipation, bloating, and/or abdominal pain, you may be undergoing dysregulation of the intestines caused by factors such as stress, which leads to high cortisol levels, menstrual irregularities and hormonal imbalances, undiagnosed food intolerances, and environmental toxins such as heavy metals.

Start regulating your digestion incrementally, mirroring the gradual accumulation of damage. Slow down and simplify your meals. Try not to combine too many varieties of protein, starches, and fats. Don't consume more than a cup of liquids prior to, during, or immediately following a meal as to not dampen your digestive fire.

Mindfully drink a cup of **BONE BROTH** (page 137), which is highly therapeutic in restoring damaged gut lining by supplying the amino acids necessary for tissue-taming collagen production, glycine for RNA and DNA synthesis for cellular repair, and glutamine for protection against mucosal breakdown in the gut. Glutamine also regulates mood, which affects digestion when imbalanced.

Among the few supplements I recommend, **HIGH QUALITY PROBIOTICS** are essential. Opt for soil-based resilient organisms that survive the early gastrointestinal tract and inoculate the intestines. If you opt for non-soil-based strains, choose a refrigerated bottle with at least 25 billion count. Further optimize the gut flora by incorporating fermented foods high in naturally occurring probiotics and enzymes that aid digestion, such as **COCONUT WATER, KEFIR, SAUERKRAUT, OLIVES, KOMBUCHA,** and **MISO** or **NATTO** if you tolerate soy products.

MAGNESIUM is necessary in over three hundred bodily reactions, one of which is digestion. It promotes balanced hormones, detoxification, and tissue regeneration.[3] The gut lining is made up of epithelial cells, so a deficiency affects sufficient digestive processing. Sufficient magnesium levels promote epithelial cell turnover and regularity, which support a healthy environment for the gut microbiome. Consume a teaspoon of magnesium powder before bed as a tea, take a bath with magnesium flakes, or spray magnesium oil for optimum absorption.

At the root of many digestive distresses is inadequate macronutrient consumption and nutrient malabsorption. When constipated, the popular hunch is to increase fiber intake while decreasing fat and protein. But

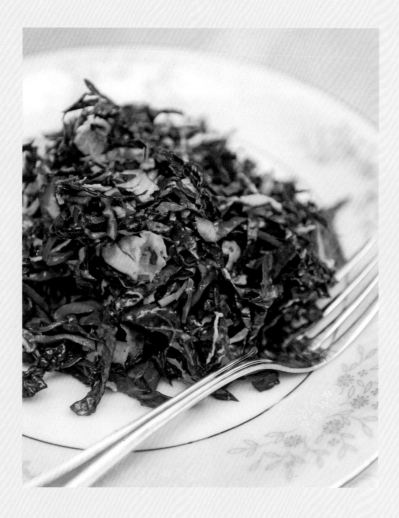

without **HEALTHY FATS** to lubricate the intestines, no amount of fiber, which can be rough on the system, will move things along. When foods cause malabsorption, it further backs digestion up. The body cannot utilize protein and vitamins in vegetables without healthy fats, which also slow the breakdown of carbohydrates into glucose that provides the steady energy you need to stave off digestion-slowing snacking.

Potty talk is inevitable on this topic—how is your posture when you're pooping? Our ancestors used to squat to poop, which positions the digestive tract for easeful excretion compared to its caving in when we sit and compress it. Try using a step stool or **SQUATTY POTTY** to raise your knees and relax the tract.

ADAPTOGENS

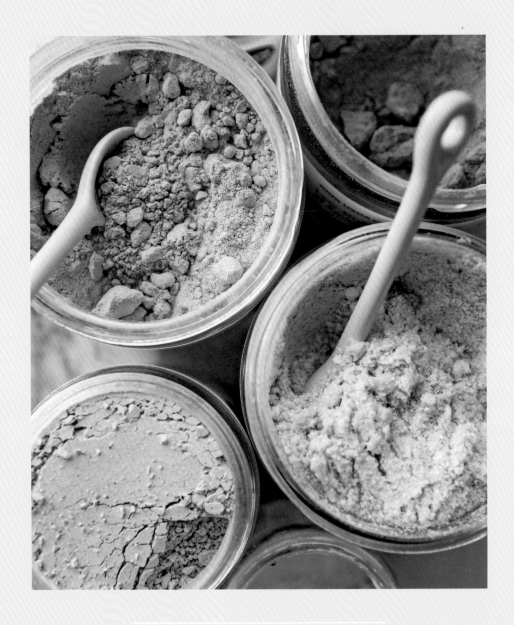

Although adaptogens are herbs and superfoods that have been used over the centuries, the term is not an ancient one. First studied in 1961 by Dr. Israel Brekhman, adaptogens were found to be safe in appropriate doses to generate resistance to environmental stressors that have negative emotional and physiological effects in the body. They normalize body functions through their amphoteric or balancing effect, treating conditions of over- or under-active systems.

They do this through the endocrine system of the HPA—hypothalamus, pituitary, and adrenal gland—axis; the nervous and immune systems; and the sympathoadrenal system. This allows for a balanced, cyclical alteration of hormone levels, immune and nervous system function, as well as stress response. Recent research has also found adaptogens have a deeper cellular effect of preventing the stress hormone cortisol from interfering with mitochondrial function. By tapping into the mitochondria (the energy factory of the body), adaptogens effectively restore efficiency to the body and allow it to heal itself.

This is what I experienced using them as healing tools for my autoimmune disorder. Through a slow, diligent, and carefully dosed inclusion of adaptogens I no longer suffer widespread joint pain and now run more than twenty miles a week. These herbs and superfoods have supported my body in its healing process and assist its harmonious functioning.

Although all adaptogens restore balance, they operate differently within the body. Certain ones like *shatavari* lubricate while others like *schizandra* dry. *Rhodiola* and cordyceps invigorate. Others tranquilize, such as *reishi* and *ashwagandha*. A quarter teaspoon—blended with tea, a smoothie, or taken in capsule form—is a gentle introductory dose (see pages 169 and 171 for two recipes). Take daily, paying close attention to how your body reacts, and adjust your personal dosage accordingly.

MUSHROOMS

REISHI: immune system strengthener; stress reliever; protection from environmental toxins and radiation

CORDYCEPS: increased athletic endurance and recovery; mental agility; increased oxygen uptake; stabilized energy levels; sexual energizer

CHAGA: antimicrobial; anti-inflammatory; immune system supporter

LION'S MANE: nervous system supporter

BOTANICALS & FOODS

ASHITABA: skin and digestive tonic; longevity

ASHWAGANDHA: tension tamer; immune system; overall strengthener

ASTRAGALUS: skin strengthener; increased metabolism; increased energy levels

HE SHOU WU: sexual and nervous system toner; blood builder; skin and hair nourisher

MUCUNA PRURIENS: mood booster; brain function enhancer; nervous system tamer

PINE POLLEN: hormone balancer; metabolism booster; increased athletic endurance; aphrodisiac

RHODIOLA: increased stamina and focus; increased oxygen flow; weight management; antioxidative

SCHIZANDRA: supports longevity, endurance, and energy

SHATAVARI: supports menstrual health

IMMUNITY

Achy groans travel down the hallways, sneezes echo in the bathroom, and coughs from labored throats abound. To get your body in balance and activate your defense system, these antimicrobial botanicals are my go-to preventative and treatment measures.

PREVENTION

OREGANO OIL is an antibacterial, antiviral, antifungal, and antihistamine that can treat infections and seasonal allergies. It's also rich in vitamins A and C, calcium, magnesium, zinc, manganese, niacin, iron, potassium, copper, and boron for preventative measures. Its main components are carvacrol, thymol, terpenes, rosmarinic, and naringin; their medicinal properties are described below.

Mix two drops of Oreganol in water and drink, preferably before bedtime, or rub a drop diluted in 2 ounces of oil such as fractionated coconut oil on the soles of the feet.

CARVACROL is a powerful antimicrobial against disease-causing microbes such as *Candida albicans*, *Staphylococcus*, *Salmonella*, *E. coli*, and *Listeria*.

THYMOL is an immune system booster and aids in tissue regeneration and flushing of toxins. It's also antifungal, which is helpful during and after the summer months with the exposure to fungal infections from swimming pools.

TERPENES not only give oregano oil its lush, pine scent but also provide antibacterial properties.

ROSMARINIC ACID is an antioxidant that is even stronger than vitamin E. It is also effective against carcinogens as well as in the treatment of allergic asthma with its antihistamine properties.

NARINGIN is a component that provides grapefruit its bitter taste, boosts the power of antioxidants such as rosmarinic, and has been shown to inhibit the growth of cancer cells.

MUSHROOMS

REISHI This mushroom provides a wide range of benefits, from suppressing the growth of cancer cells to anti-inflammatory uses for Alzheimer's and Parkinson's. It is deeply healing for the respiratory and circulatory systems as it strengthens the lungs and improves blood and oxygen flow to the heart.

CORDYCEPS Technically a fungi, cordyceps has a long history of medicinal use. It is considered a potent yang tonic that oxygenates the body, stimulates the immune system, protects against free radical damage, and tones the muscles of the organs for optimum function.

TURKEY TAIL This common mushroom, which looks a lot like a turkey tail, targets chronic illnesses and cancer cells, aids in the regeneration of bone marrow, and is a strong antioxidant.

TREATMENT

VITAMIN D T-cells are an essential aspect of our immune system. To be effective, they require adequate levels of vitamin D in the body. The sun is the optimal source of natural vitamin D and only ten minutes of exposure sans sunscreen can give us our daily requirement. During the darker, colder months of autumn and winter, boost the body with food sources high in vitamin D such as cod liver oil, organic, local, pasture-raised eggs, grass-fed butter or ghee, shiitake mushrooms, and fatty fish such as salmon or sardines. Supplements are also beneficial in liquid form, but be careful of overdosing. Vitamin D is fat-soluble, which means that its excess will be stored in fat tissue, where it can accumulate and become toxic. It comes in two forms: vitamin D2 and D3. The latter is the more readily metabolized form of vitamin D, so much so that it yields "the production of unique biologically active metabolites."[4] The Premier Research version is the best out there as it's not suspended in inflammatory vegetable oils and/or artificial flavorings like most other brands.

ALLIUMS such as garlic and onions are antibacterial. They can be taken orally and also applied topically for issues such as a stye or cold sore that can come along with a compromised immune system. After cutting a clove of garlic in half, let it sit for 15 minutes, then rub the cut side of the clove directly on the stye or cold sore. Other alliums are also powerful in preventing and reducing the duration of colds and flu. Traditional healers often recommend supplementing with a concoction called Fire Cider in times of high exposure to germs—I love Rosemary Gladstar's recipe. You can also make a tonic by adding 2 cloves crushed garlic to 2 ounces apple cider vinegar to chug. Placing a handful of garlic cloves in boiling water and inhaling its vapors is also great for combating nasal congestion.

TURMERIC is a blood and liver purifier, anti-inflammatory, tissue regenerating, and lymph-draining. It heals the immune system by decreasing the cytokines that block the appropriate drainage of the lymphatic system and immune response. Mix ¼ teaspoon of tumeric powder with 1 teaspoon each of apple cider vinegar and antimicrobial Manuka honey in ¼ cup water with a dash of black pepper. Enjoy knocking it back like a shot.

PROBIOTICS and **FERMENTED FOODS** Our gut is considered our "second brain," impacting everything from energy levels to metabolism to the condition of our skin. Doubling your probiotic supplement dosage to include both morning and night while increasing your consumption of fermented foods such as sauerkraut, coconut kefir, kombucha, and other cultured foods will increase good bacteria to activate the immune system.

ELDERBERRY A staple component of many naturopathic cold and flu medications, elderberry is a strong inhibitor of the growth of viral infections and at shortening their duration. Take a tincture (page 40) at the first sign of illness.

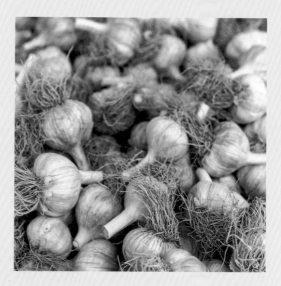

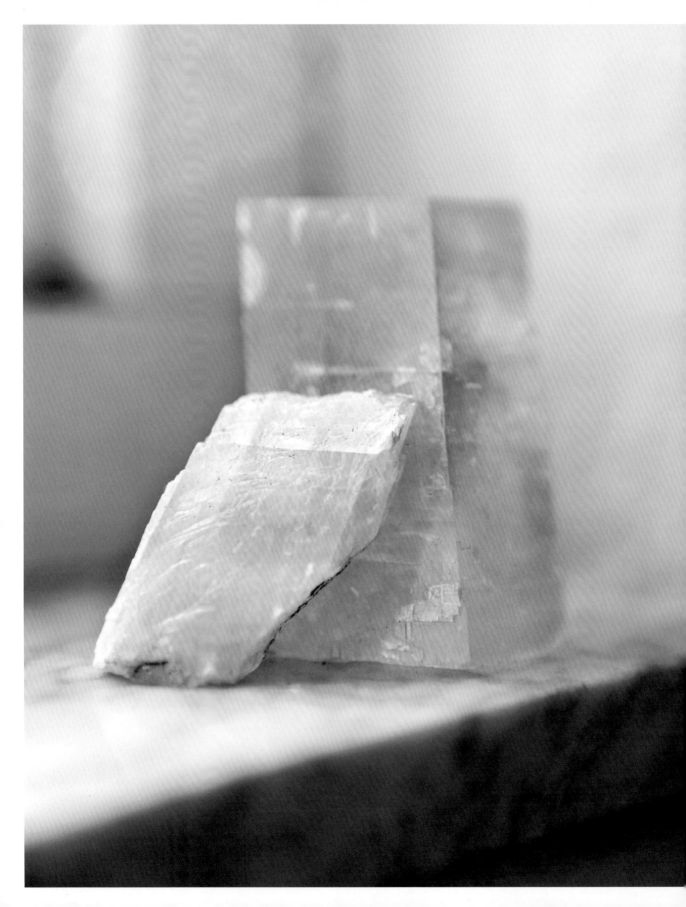

BREATHWORK

Observe your breath and you'll most likely discover its shallowness. The breath, although automatic, can also be controlled. An **AWARE BREATH** can be a bridge to the vastness of an unconscious, open mind by softening our habitual responses or held emotions. When we cultivate our knowledge of breathing, we can free up ideas or emotions stored away in our consciousness.

Breathwork should not be a forcing of a **RHYTHM** that is unnatural for your body. It's not a superimposed cycle of breathing that burdens our own. Rather, it's a **PRACTICE** to return your breath to its own cadence without the threat of tension. The majority of stress is contained within the chest, which is both the seat of shallow breathing and action. When we're working, it's natural for the breath to be higher in location than when at rest. We cannot expect nor should we move our breath into the abdomen, away from the conscious action within the chest. Aware, abdominal breathing generates a slower meditative or restful mode. Many people believe that they should always breathe from **THE BELLY**. There is a time and place for a quiet state—we cannot expect to do our jobs in a peaceful trance. So, higher breathing has its purpose, but it's also a seat of tension.

This is especially the case for those who identify as women, with the social pressure and identity oppression through the breasts. The chest is also where we nonverbally signify ourselves and the throne in which the ego sits. When we grapple with issues of self-identity, self-doubt, sexuality, trust, and our voice, we cave into our chest and hinder our breathing. Breathwork allows us to reclaim our *selves* through our breath and bodies. As tight shoulders loosen and posture is restored, so is our sense of self. Our life force—*prana* in ayurveda and *qi* in TCM—is restored, creating a channel of energy.

To get started, sit comfortably or lie down on the floor with closed eyes. Tune into your body and notice where you feel movement as you breathe. Breathe in and out through the nose, slowly relaxing and triggering your natural rhythm.

Allow your breath to suffuse into these areas and ease tension. Draw out your exhales slowly and gently. This balances the oxygen uptake and restores the body's sympathetic and parasympathetic nervous systems. Create a natural respiratory cycle to equalize your breath into relaxation. Once you establish your natural smooth rhythm, place your hand on your abdomen and begin to breathe into it. Feel the gentle rise and fall. Reflect this softening in other body parts starting from the head—loosen your jaw, eyelids, eyebrows—and down to your toes until you've released bodily tensions. Practice for at least ten minutes every day.

ENERGY MEDICINE

Three anthropologists and a doctor are standing by a river when they hear the cries of a drowning man. The doctor jumps in the river and resuscitates him. Another one floats by shortly afterward and again, he attempts resuscitation. More bodies follow. It finally occurs to one of the anthropologists to go upstream and investigate the cause, while another searches for cautionary clues, and the third stays to assist the doctor-patient relationship.

This story illustrates the Newtonian medical system that we navigate, which offers drugs and surgery only after illness strikes. The body is viewed as a container of organs rather than a dynamic system.

Rather than taking a narrow cause-and-effect approach to illness, Energy Medicine shifts the focus to optimizing health. It does this by shifting the conventional medicine focus on the biochemistry of cells and organs to the energy fields of the body. When the flow of energy is optimal in these fields, they have the potential to aid in the reparation of the body. The practices of Energy Medicine, such as the following Daily Rituals, shift impaired energy patterns to revive the physical body and psyche. In doing so, Energy Medicine simultaneously heals the body from illnesses and equips it to overcome future challenges by reintegrating the body, mind, and spirit.

All biological processes are energetic at their foundation—*energy is all there is*. If energy is shifted, the energetic intelligence independent of the mind has to respond. Every component from atom and molecule to the organs vibrates in our bodies, which determines our health. By restoring each component's energetic state, we restore vitality and optimal function.

DAILY RITUALS

THE THREE THUMPS restores energy and lymphatic flow. Use your fingers to tap on the points below for twenty seconds each as you take deep breaths to oxygenate them.

- **K-27** is the tender spot below the collarbone, near the u-shape on the upper corner of the upper breastbone.

- **The Thymus** is located at the center of the sternum.

- **The Neurolymphatic Spleen** points are below the breasts on the second rib.

THE CROSS CRAWL balances the hemispheres of the brain and overall body coordination.

Stand and begin a kind of exaggerated march as you raise your right arm and left leg on an inhale, lower the right arm and left leg as you exhale, raise your left arm and right leg on an inhale, lower the left arm and right leg as you exhale. Repeat for at least one minute.

THE HOOK UP clears the auric field and residual stuck energy. Place one middle finger on the point between the eyebrows (your third eye) and the other middle finger on the navel. Gently press in and up for a minute on both points, breathing deeply.

THE NEUROVASCULAR HOLD is an energetic remedy for dispelling tension or the blues. This practice is the evolutionary equivalent of running away from danger, providing an antidote to calm the brain away from thinking of looming deadlines or overwhelming to-do lists. Place your thumbs on your temples and lay your fingers across your forehead. Press gently for three minutes as you breathe deeply from the abdomen.

Complete your daily rituals with the energy-protective **ZIP UP** by slowly moving your hands from the base of your pubic bone up to your mouth, as if zipping your energy up. Repeat three times.

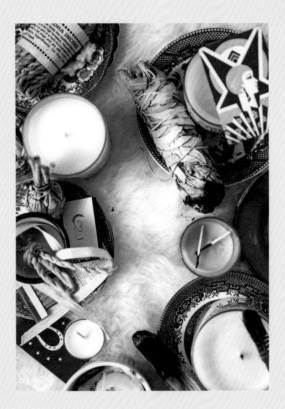

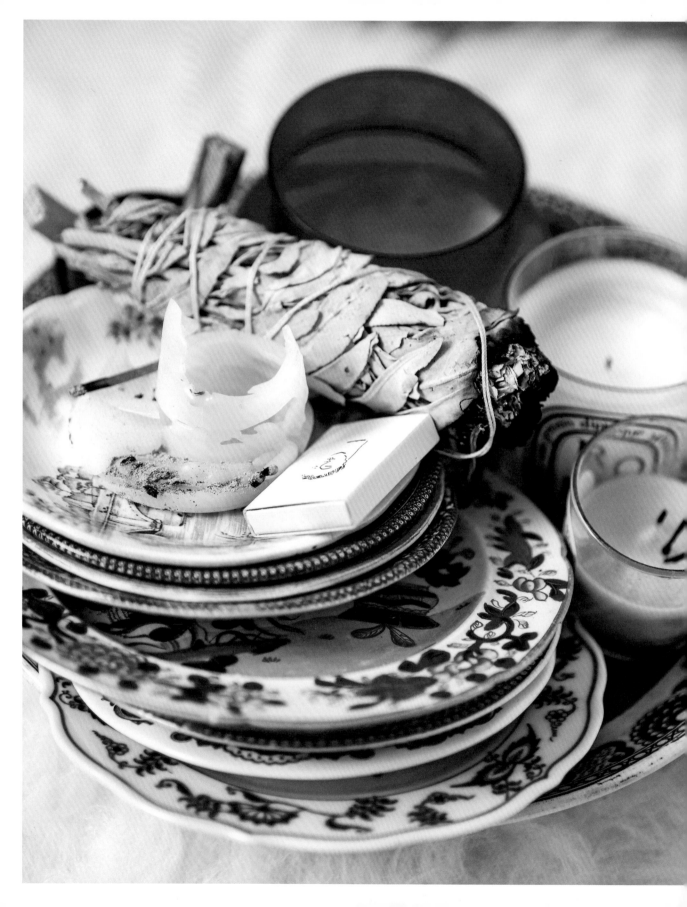

MEDITATIVE MANTRAS

Even with years of meditation practice, it can be a task to sit down on your cushion. On days in which we are threatened by the traffic jams of our mind, mantras can cut through the onslaught of thoughts ranging from the dirty dishes in the sink to a dirty joke. A **MANTRA** is a sound or word that functions as a vehicle to bring the mind into a still-point of focus, creating a subtle space for a physiological release of tension.

There are a variety of meditative mantras that can be chanted, repeated over rosary beads, or spoken silently. The **AYURVEDIC MANTRAS** below supply the body with sounds that are energetically aligned with our specific constitution (see page 54 for more on doshas)—the vibrations of the mantra balances an erratic dosha, or physical constitution, bringing the subtle body to homeostasis. The mantras can be repeated for as long as necessary.

For the easily aggravated **VATA** dosha, the soothing mantra of SHRIM can be repeated. This mantra will induce a sense of purpose, which can easily be lost within the over-committed vata mind. It can also be utilized to generate prosperity, increase health, and creative flow.

Mantras should not be repeated for too long or too loud by vata constitutions as this can deplete the already fragile levels of energy. If you prefer chanting out loud, balance this by doing it out loud for a few minutes then continuing mentally. HOOM and AUM are also other mantras that can bring softness into the rigid state of vata.

The mantra best aligned with **PITTA** is RAM, which is the mantra of Truth. Pitta constitutions need mantras that bring a sense of cooling as they tend to run hot and irritated, which can be further aggravated when trying to drop into meditation. Other calming mantras are SHRIM, AUM, and SHAM.

KAPHA constitutions greatly benefit from chanting as it generates warmth and stimulation for their sluggish tendencies, especially when out of balance. The mantra HRIM allows for the purification and cleansing of this constitution while supplying it with a stream of energy. Other mantras that provide activation for kapha individuals are HOOM and AUM.

◈

TAMING ANXIETY & PAIN

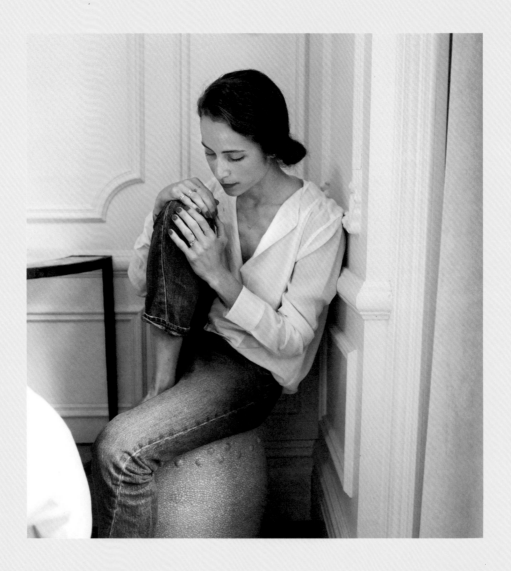

When self-care is neglected like a forgotten pair of socks, it paves the way for an inflammatory response. Pathways of stress reaction are activated in efforts to combat the multitude of pressures that we navigate physically, emotionally, chemically, and environmentally. These are all factors which, if unmanaged, cyclically cause elevated stress levels. Untamed anxiety disrupts hormone levels, causing physical symptoms of menstrual irregularities. Toxic ingredients in products we put on our bodies, such as **ALUMINUM** in deodorants, can bioaccumulate to cause a host of stress-induced ailments.

Managing both emotional and physical pain requires caring for how we physically and emotionally feed our bodies. We must process our thoughts, feelings, and emotions for proper flow of energy or **PRANA**. Unprocessed or **UNCONTAINED EMOTIONS** get stored in our physical tissues and create energetic blockages. You can release these emotions by understanding uncontained emotions (page 100), **MEDITATING, SPEAKING WITH A THERAPIST, ART THERAPY**, or **JOURNALING**.

SEASONAL CHANGES are also a dominant factor in mood changes. The waning sun and decreased sunlight cause biochemical imbalances in the brain. Our **INTERNAL CIRCADIAN RHYTHM** and **MELATONIN PRODUCTION**, which regulate a range of functions from sleep to hormones, shift with the seasons. This fluctuation leads to symptoms including fatigue, brain fog, irritability, lack of concentration, decreased libido, and even depression. As melatonin is a hormone, these seasonal reactions can cause a plethora of other hormonal imbalances when untamed, such as menstrual irregularities, digestive distress, and consequential skin breakouts.

MOOD REGULATORS

LIGHT THERAPY is a helpful tool for regulating environmental stressors. It simulates sunlight for brief periods of time daily to harmonize circadian rhythm and consequently boost mood.

One of the most critical vitamins in mood regulation is vitamin D, which many people are deficient in no matter the season. Supplementation is especially necessary during the darker months, but not all vitamin D is created equal. Avoid vitamin D2 and opt for hexane-free vitamin D3 suspended in an additive-free base.

The **OMEGA-3 FATTY ACIDS** in wild-caught seafood, raw and sprouted nuts and seeds, and avocados heighten the function of neural tracks which regulate mood. Incorporate plant-based options such as complete protein hemp seeds, raw oysters high in mood-boosting zinc, or wild-caught salmon.

Proper forms of **B VITAMINS** play a critical role in neurological functions. Opt for bioavailable or easily absorbable lypospheric or at least end-chain form B vitamin complex that is not derived from coal tar. The top food sources are shellfish, organ meats, wild-caught fish, grass-fed beef, and pastured eggs.

WARM BATHS with epsom salt, mustard powder, fresh grated ginger, apple cider vinegar, or baking soda relax muscle constriction which can help release physical and emotional pain. Essential oils of lavender, frankincense, chamomile, bergamot, and vetiver tame anxiety while black cumin, clove, and oregano target physical inflammation. Dilute these in a carrier oil and massage. Ready-made options include Narayan Balm or White Flower Balm.

Address emotional pathways with **FLOWER REMEDIES** such as Mimulus and Aspen for fear, Red Chestnut for worrying about others, Elm for feeling overwhelmed, and White Chestnut for unwanted thoughts or judgements.

ENERGETIC PROTECTION

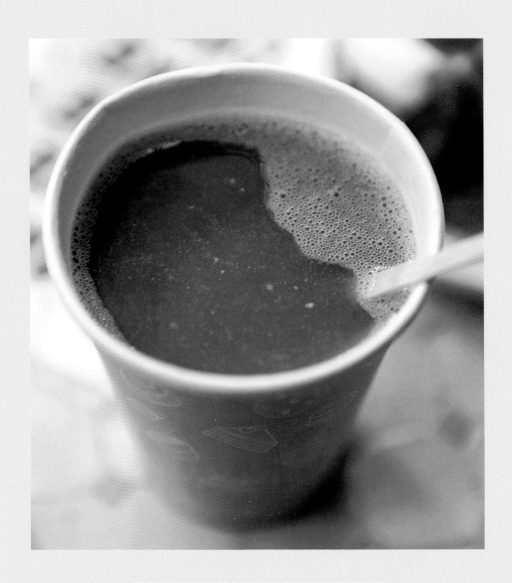

I remember how back in high school, I used to sleep with my cell phone right next to my pillow awaiting cryptic text messages of young love. But love wasn't the only naïve part of that situation—so was keeping my phone right near my head.

Technological gadgets of all kinds emit electromagnetic radiation (EMF) which can increase the risk of a brain cancer[5] and lower sperm motility by 8 percent, among other harmful effects.[6] To decrease daily EMF exposure, it is therefore crucial to keep gadgets away from our bodies during sleep when we don't need them. If you can't move your phone away from your bedroom or use it as an alarm, put your phone on airplane mode. Turn off and unplug anything electrical in your room as well that is unnecessary until the morning, such as computers.

During the day, try to be more mindful of your phone usage by keeping some physical and mental distance. When speaking on the phone, either speak on speaker or use headphones to reduce EMF exposure. Turn off your phone when possible, since no radiation is emitted when it's off. If you take the metro, put it on **AIRPLANE MODE** or turn it off during your ride since there's usually no signal anyway and EMF increases significantly when your phone is desperately searching for it. Radiation also increases when Bluetooth is on, so turn it off when unnecessary. There are even radiation-protective cases, such as **SILVERSHIELD** or **PONG** for phones and **DEFENDERSHIELD** for laptops.

Additionally, we can protect ourselves through shielding our bodies with **HIGH-VIBRATION FOODS** and **EARTHY ELEMENTS**. Eating foods that nourish the nervous system boosts the body's primal shield—the brain—against EMFs. Bone broth (page 137), sea vegetables such as chlorella and spirulina, and fermented or cultured foods such as sauerkraut (page 178) all provide cellular and detoxification support. Consume these daily if possible.

An **EMF-PROTECTIVE DIET** also includes eating high ORAC or antioxidant foods, such as turmeric, matcha green tea, and wild berries. Flushing our systems with cruciferous vegetables—organic when and if possible—such as broccoli, cabbage, daikon, and cauliflower also balances the system with necessary antioxidants and sulfur. Sulfur is a necessary nutrient for proper mitochondrial function, which regulates the entire body's energy assimilation. Herbs such as parsley, cilantro, and holy basil are also supportive.

For external protection, keep crystals such as **BLACK TOURMALINE**, **AMAZONITE**, **LEPIDOLITE**, or **SODALITE** near your technological devices and bedside table near your phone at night. Himalayan pink salt lamps in bedrooms or in the office also provide protection against EMF.

Still, the most effective way to detoxify our bodies and our minds of EMF radiation is to consciously separate ourselves from technology. For me, this usually means a barefoot walk outside. Hikes, walks, or being outside can shift the perspective from the narrow parameters of our gadgets out into the grandness of life. It's easy to spiral down the rabbit hole of seeing life through the perfect tableaux of social media. We are swept into endless scrolls and networks of accounts through which we compare our own selves and work, unaware of what the lives of others truly entail. Unplugging from social media and our phones liberates us from these comparative stories. Go outside instead and allow yourself to reconnect to your external and internal authentic nature, sinking back to your roots.

UTILIZING CRYSTALS

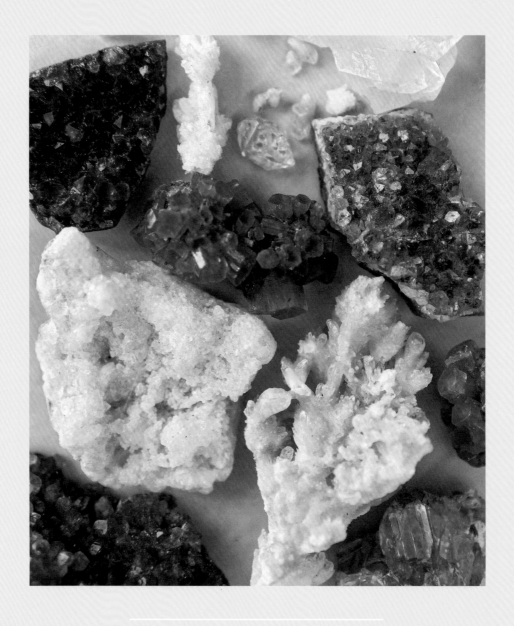

Quartz: master healer

Green Aventurine: abundance

Amethyst: anti-anxiety

Moonstone & Lapis Lazuli: creativity and intuition

Black Tourmaline: protection

Tiger's Eye: mental clarity

Rose Quartz: love

Ruby: vitality

Crystals are underground mineral formations often developing over thousands of years. Their repeating chemical compositions invest them with certain energetic properties. This allows crystals to balance energies of the physical and etheric bodies, affecting internal and external relationships. In simple yet powerful terms, crystals are containers of energy that affect our individual vibrational frequencies.

Their unique structure also acts as a kind of memory that allows them to retain the energy or wishes of their owner. For instance, holding a rose quartz with the intention of increasing self-love will program it to imbue this energy into your surroundings. However, crystals can also retain negative energies, so it's important to cleanse crystals regularly. Although there are various ways to cleanse crystals, such as submerging them in salt or sea water and burying them in the ground for a few days, I find

that leaving crystals out on New and Full Moons not only cleanses the crystals but also imbues them with the energies of that particular moon phase.

CRYSTAL THERAPY is the placement of certain crystals on appropriate parts of the body that align with the seven chakras—colorful centers of subtle energy running through the center of the torso—to expel disease. This is why crystals of specific colors such as purple amethyst, aligned with the mind center of the chakras, aid in relaxation.

COLOR can be an intuitive guide for picking the crystal that will best serve you. I suggest going to a crystal shop instead of shopping online to let your senses find what energetically calls to you. You might feel a pull toward a certain crystal and, reading of its properties, find that it aids the exact struggles you've been facing.

SHAPES also affect the energetic properties of crystals. Single terminated wands are effective for cleansing energy; clusters and chunks enhance the energy of a room; cut crystals aid in meditation; and tumblestones are great to carry around in the pocket throughout the day.

HEALING GRID

When you face the major point of a crystal away from an imbalanced area , it will remove the problematic energy, while facing that point toward an imbalanced area will recharge it. A crystal guidebook can help you choose calming crystals for the former and energizing crystals for the latter.

Use four amethyst points to quell bodily pain. Lie down. Place one on each collar bone at the base of the throat facing up toward the head; another on the middle of the forehead facing up; and the last above the crown of the head facing up. Take a nap for at least 15 minutes.

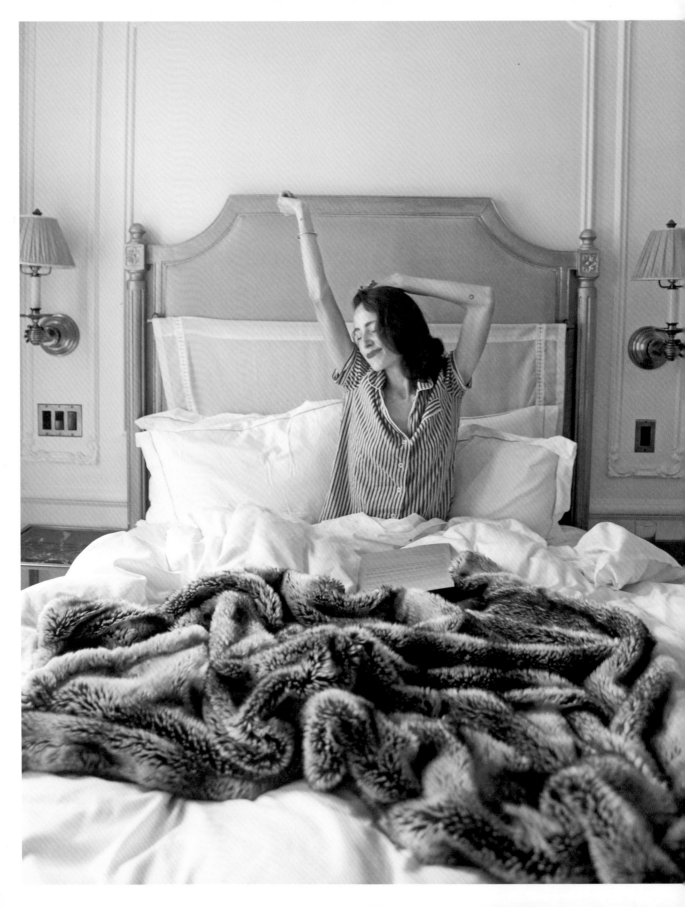

HACKING SLEEP

We spend on average a third of our life in bed. The following is a guide to biohacking your brain and body into sweeter slumbers, from moonlit rituals to bedside staples.

Eating a heavy meal, especially close to your bedtime, can wreak havoc on your sleep cycle. The body rests most optimally when dinner has been digested well, so allow three hours between dinner and bedtime. Try to limit alcohol consumption when accompanying a light dinner—breakfast and lunch should be your main sources of fuel. Cut out caffeine after 2 P.M., as its effects can carry through the evening and cause difficulty falling asleep.

As with late dinners, rigorous exercise too close to your bedtime can disrupt the sleep cycle, although some people claim to rest better with an evening workout. Experiment with what feels right for your body. Alternatively, try a **YIN YOGA** routine instead, which can pacify vata qualities—the ayurvedic constitution primarily responsible for our irritability and tensions—that emerge during times of high stress.

As much as we aspire to turn off our computers in the evening, most of us are unable to minimize our screen time. A way to hack into the digital rabbit hole is to use **F.LUX SOFTWARE**, which is designed to adjust your screen's brightness according to the time of day. Specifically, the software adjusts the levels of blue light which, according to research, are the most disruptive to melatonin levels. These days, most smartphones have a night shift option built in, which uses the clock and geolocation to adjust the lighting of your phone.

A room that is completely dark—so much so that if you raised your hand you would not be able to see it—is essential for a good night's sleep. To get your room to this level of darkness, cover your windows with blackout curtains and wear a **SILK EYE MASK**, which has the additional benefit of providing moisture balance for the skin.

Regulating the body's temperature through a warm bath is a quick way to induce sleepiness as the body shifts itself to cooler temperatures. Add in **EPSOM SALT** or **MUSTARD POWDER** for achy, tired joints.

If you cannot keep your monkey mind jumping from one thought to another, have a journal nearby to jot down to-do or gratitude lists. Keeping a diary for journaling the day is also a calming way to take a step back from the daily occurrences, see the big picture, celebrate or contemplate, and surrender.

A cup of **HERBAL TEA** is another way to prepare the body for sleep. Choosing the right, targeted tea blend can also provide added benefits. Try detoxifying single-herb varieties like nettle leaf, raspberry leaf, dandelion root, marshmallow root, or slippery elm, all of which either support the liver, digestion, or reproductive system to expel built-up toxins in the morning.

And finally, a spoonful of **RAW HONEY** in the evening can help ease you into sweet slumber. The medicinal use of honeybee products (apitherapy) and true raw, unfiltered honey, which is filled with beeswax, pollen, and propolis, provides the body with stick-to-the-bones medicinal comfort.

HANGOVER CURES

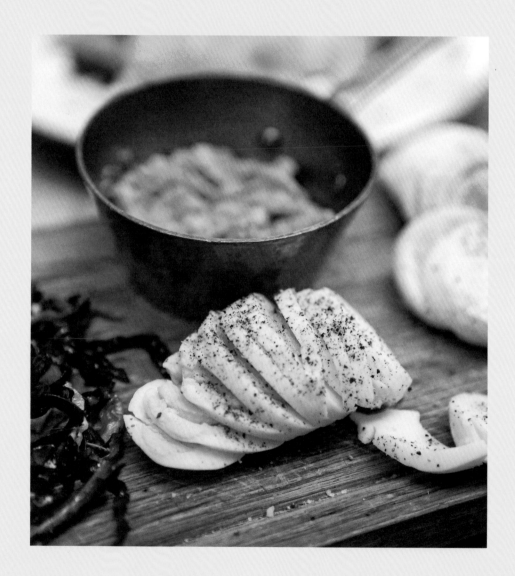

Prevention precedes treatment for ailments and is key especially when it comes to alcohol consumption. When the body is prepared and alcohol is consciously consumed, hangovers can generally be avoided.

Before heading out for drinks, increase your **WATER INTAKE** to combat the dehydrating effect. Alcohol also depletes levels of B vitamins, so supplementing with a higher-absorptive liquid B vitamin complex will restore the system and boost metabolic function. **MILK THISTLE** is another supplement which provides metabolic and liver protection with antioxidants silymarin and silybum.

Native American medicine holds that eating a handful of **RAW ALMONDS** can provide a protective threshold for a hangover. In traditional West African medicine, a similar preventative recommends eating peanut butter before imbibing. I recommend almonds over the inflammatory peanut. The protein in nuts provides satiation and balances blood sugar levels that alcohol spikes, while the healthy fats protect the liver from toxins.

When you are consuming alcohol, try not to mix too many drinks, such as a figurative cocktail of wine, shots, and mixed drinks; **REMAIN SIMPLE** and stick to the drinks that your body tolerates well. Take the time to enjoy each drink, allow your body to absorb it, and hydrate adequately in between glasses.

When you're back from a night out, eat a **BANANA**. The potassium will replenish electrolytes and the magnesium will restore proper muscle function, which will increase blood flow to prevent headaches. The simple sugars fructose and glucose will also provide the body with easily assimilable energy to metabolize alcohol and balance the energy source of glycogen levels to "burn the alcohol faster."[7]

RAW HONEY is another option before bed according the Royal Society of Chemistry. The fructose similarly aids in the processing of alcohol as it stabilizes blood glucose and replenishes glycogen, which the liver uses to restore itself during sleep. The added live enzymes also support digestive breakdown of alcoholic toxins, such as additives, coloring, preservatives, and even mold. Incorporate a teaspoon before bed for sweet slumber.

Drinking **WARM WATER WITH LEMON** as soon as you wake up will rehydrate, cleanse the liver, and increase pH levels from the acidity caused by alcohol. In the case of nausea, make ginger tea by boiling an inch of fresh ginger or ½ teaspoon of dried ginger in 2 cups of water. This will also aid in soothing digestion and nutrient assimilation. Bone broth is also an easily digested source of protein and replenisher of lost electrolytes.

A breakfast of **EGGS** will provide cysteine, which is an amino acid found to further assist in the digestion of toxins found in alcohol.[8] Cook the eggs in coconut oil, which contains anti-inflammatory and antimicrobial properties to avoid over-the-counter pain killers and combat the oxidative state caused by drinking. The healthy saturated fats will also stimulate digestion and bowel movement for detoxification.

Activating the body's own healing system through **ACUPRESSURE POINTS** can also relieve symptoms. Stimulating the reflex point located on the outer edge of the right foot, halfway between the little toe and the middle of the foot, will assist in cleansing the liver and alleviate headaches.

SENSUAL SEDUCTION

The impoverished conditions of our modern sexuality are as laughable as the song this section gets its title from. Our bedrooms are often lit by smartphones rather than romantic candles, but it's not merely an aesthetic disconnect at play here—we are disconnected from our beliefs and our bodies.

Many of us preach the use of non-toxic products but don't consider what we use between the sheets. Our standards for natural ingredients often go down like a one-night stand when it comes to sex. Most condoms and lubricants on the market contain carcinogenic and hormone-disrupting chemicals like nitrosamines and petrochemicals that disrupt the vaginal ecosystem, causing issues such as bacterial overgrowth. They also contain parabens and glycerin, which can cause significant cellular damage and increase the risk for contracting STIs or STDs. The good news is there are alternative options that can protect and pleasure the body.

However, before we turn down the sheets, let us start by asking ourselves how we are connecting to our own sexuality. In other words, what is your relationship to your own genitalia? Are you protective of them? Or have you disconnected them from the rest of your body? When was the last time you examined your genitalia? Do you guard your own self against this area but permit others the right to touch it? Many women experience shame or discomfort looking at or touching their own genitalia, but

Natural Alternatives for Condoms & Lubricants

- **Sustain Natural condoms:** Made without nitrosamines, these condoms are fair trade, vegan, and sustainable.

- **Coconut oil:** Make sure to use it as a lubricant with non-latex condoms since oil-based lubricants will degrade latex.

- **Good Clean Love:** Made from safe and simple ingredients such as aloe vera, this vegan lubricant comes in "naked" as well as cinnamon vanilla flavors.

- **Sylk:** This lubricant is derived from New Zealand kiwifruit extract and contains no harsh chemicals, hormones, or animal products.

allow others such as a doctor or a partner to do so. If you fall into this category, you might want to think about your relationship to your genitalia and where you learned your sexual associations.

You can begin to explore this by looking at your vagina with a mirror. You might feel discomfort by the mere thought or act of this—consider why you have this response. Use a full-length mirror to visually and psychologically reconnect your vagina to the rest of your body. Look at and feel your vagina. Examine the labia, your clitoris, contract and release your muscles, observe the sensations that ensue.

Next, lie down in a comfortable area to perform some pelvic exercises. Close your eyes and surrender any tension to the ground. Slowly breathe deeply from the abdomen, imagining the pelvis filling with a cleansing inhale and releasing tension with an exhale out through your vagina. After a few cycles, notice how your vagina and body feel.

Now focus on your vaginal muscles. In yogic traditions, this area holds the seat of our most powerful energy or *kundalini*. When stimulated through awareness and exercise, the energy held can be released up through the spine and activate higher energy channels. To engage this center, simply "clench" your pubic muscles as if trying to hold in urine. Then release. Repeat twenty times daily for increased tone and flexibility for sex, pregnancy, and childbirth.

MENSTRUAL
MANAGEMENT

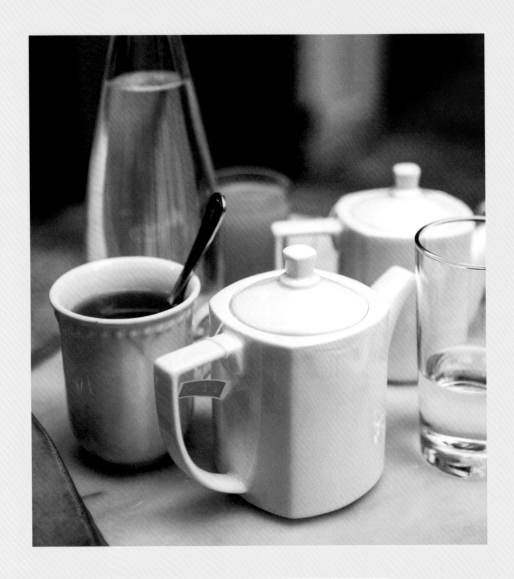

I got my period at the tender age of nine and lost it shortly after when I developed anorexia at age eleven. I was emotionally traumatized by the one-night notice of moving from Turkey to the United States. In the ensuing anxiety, I was left unequipped with anything but creating a control system of disordered eating. This created further emotional—and an additional level of physiological—trauma to my body.

I eventually restored my weight and consequently my period until a relapse in college, where I lost it again for over three years.

I share this abridged version of my journey to illustrate how menstruation is not merely a physiological mechanism. It's governed by the three bodies—physical, emotional, and spiritual—which can cause menstrual imbalance if any one of them is out of sync. Managing menstruation requires conscious awareness of what we feed ourselves emotionally, materially, and spiritually.

To regulate hormones, incorporate the following to your regimen and practice patience.

Avoid **INFLAMMATORY FOODS** that aggravate hormones, such as dairy products, grains, refined sugars, and vegetable oils. Reduce your caffeine intake as it dehydrates the fluid retentive body and can cause breast tenderness. Instead, focus on increasing healthy fats, such as ghee—technically dairy but contains very little milk protein—which has fat-soluble vitamins and cholesterol that are the metabolic building blocks for sex hormones. Insulin spikes from refined carbohydrates and sugar aggravate estrogen dominance that often cause menstrual symptoms. Incorporating a healthy balance for stable blood sugar levels is the fastest way to signal the endocrine system that it's supported. Focus on **NUTRIENT-DENSE** and easily assimilated foods like bone broth as well as its hydrolyzed components collagen and gelatin (page 137), grass-fed meats or sprouted nuts and seeds, healthy fats, and dark, leafy green vegetables to rebuild the blood.

Magnesium is also necessary for insulin sensitivity as well as estrogen and glucose metabolism for proper hormone function. When supplemented, it can harmonize estrogen levels and relieve symptoms like muscle cramping. Incorporate 250 mg twice daily for symptom relief or prevention before your period.

In any menstrual disorder, regulating blood flow is critical. Angelica, peony, he shou wu, and rehmannia root are **CHINESE HERBS** that nourish the blood and reduce menstrual symptoms. As each herb can have a different effect according to levels of hormonal imbalance, please consult a health practitioner as always before consuming them. **MACA**, highlighted on page 143, is a safer option as it's a root, often ground into powder. Begin by incorporating a teaspoon daily, especially for estrogen dominance. **ASHITABA** builds the blood, replenishes vitamin B, and supports digestion that can go awry during menstruation.

For **TENDER BREASTS**, create a warm compress with a drop each of juniper berry and cypress essential oils. A warm bath with these oils also eases water retention—use four drops of each.

Dilute four drops of either lavender, peppermint, geranium, or sweet marjoram per two ounces of carrier oil to rub on neck and shoulders for **HEADACHE RELIEF**; and on the abdomen or lower back as a warm compress for **CRAMPS**.

Place a warm compress on the lower abdomen with two drops of either cypress, frankincense, or geranium for **MILD BLEEDING**, and basil, clary sage, or juniper berry for **HEAVY BLEEDING**.

HERBAL TINCTURES

A tincture is a liquid herbal preparation that extracts healing alkaloids, essential oils, minerals, and gly-cosides into a solvent base. This base is often high-proof alcohol such as vodka but can also include alcohol-free versions of vegetable glycerin and apple cider vinegar although these formulations are less effective at extracting medicinal benefits. If you are managing a celiac diagnosis, make sure that your alcohol is not grain-based. Opt for grape- or potato-based vodka. By preserving herbs as a tinc-ture, they are rendered more effective and can last as long as ten years. It's a great option for children especially as they can be simply dissolved in water or applied externally.

EQUIPMENT

80 proof or higher consumable alcohol (such as vodka) or raw apple cider vinegar

Dried herb of your choice (page 41)

16-ounce glass container with tight-fitting lid

Fine strainer

Cotton cheesecloth

Measuring cup

Funnel

Amber or cobalt vials with dropper for storage of prepared tincture

NOTE *High-proof alcohol with dry rather than fresh herbs prevent bacterial contamination and mildewing.*

Once you've chosen your menstruum or solvent, fill a quarter* of your container with the dried herb of your choice. The alcohol will reconstitute it as the plant matter swells. Fill the rest of the container with your menstruum, stir to incorpo-rate, then securely tighten the lid. Label and date your container then store in a cool, dark area. In the first week, shake the container daily to incorporate the herbs well. Afterward, let it sit for five more weeks to total a month-and-a-half of steeping.

Once you are done steeping, prepare for extraction by placing a strainer lined with a layer of cheesecloth over a measuring cup. Pour the contents of the tincture through the strainer then squeeze remaining liquid out of the cloth.

Place the funnel into your storage vial and pour in the tincture. Label the bottle and store in a dark place.

NOTE *Although generally the ratio of herb to menstruum is 1:4, research your selected plant as there are exceptions for certain stronger plants.*

HERB OPTIONS

ASTRAGALUS ROOT: immune system

DANDELION ROOT: liver support; detoxifier; diuretic; menstrual support

BURDOCK ROOT: liver, bladder, blood, and skin tonic

CHAMOMILE OR LEMON BALM: emotional support

DAMIANA: aphrodisiac

GINSENG: immune system; brain fog; lethargy; mild depression

LICORICE ROOT: digestive; nausea; glandular tonic; hypothyroidic depression

NETTLES: malnourishment; fatigue; allergies

SLIPPERY ELM: digestive

MARSHMALLOW ROOT: digestive

GINGER: digestive

RASPBERRY LEAF: antispasmodic for menstrual or muscle cramps; hormone balance; heavy menstruation

ST. JOHN'S WORT: moderate depression; anxiety

YARROW: stimulates or increases menstrual flow for irregular or absent periods

SAGE: stimulates or increases menstrual flow for irregular or absent periods

ROSEMARY: stimulates or increases menstrual flow for irregular or absent periods

MOTHERWORT: stimulates or increases menstrual flow for irregular or absent periods

VALERIAN: insomnia; menstrual cramps

VITEX BERRY: hormone balance; heavy menstruation

WHITE WILLOW BARK: painkiller; fever reducer; anti-inflammatory; sedative

WILD LETTUCE: painkiller; fever reducer; anti-inflammatory; sedative

MEADOWSWEET: painkiller; fever reducer; anti-inflammatory; sedative

HERBAL
FIRST AID KIT

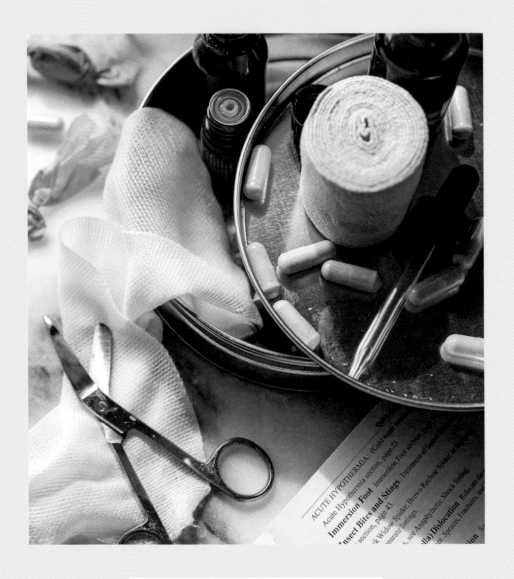

First aid kits are often stocked with staples like bandages and surgical tapes, but also chemically derived and toxic conventional preparations. Anti-inflammatory drugs (NSAIDs) such as ibuprofen not only contain toxic fillers but certain types can increase cardiovascular disease risk by up to 63 percent.[9]

We must recognize inflammation as a natural reaction for an injured or infected body. It triggers a series of biochemical responses to fight off foreign bodies. Anti-inflammatory drugs do not necessarily rid the body of the issue but rather provide temporary relief. They are also processed, foreign substances that further tax an already expended body. The body could instead use this energy to fight infection or injury with natural substances that do not interfere with its own immune responses.

ACTIVATED CHARCOAL and **BENTONITE CLAY** are antidotes mainly for food poisoning but also for digestive ailments including intestinal infections, ingestion of toxins, vomiting, and diarrhea. Take 4 activated charcoal tablets or 1 teaspoon of bentonite clay every hour 3 to 4 times per day or until symptoms subside. Make sure to increase water intake as they are dehydrating.

NOTE *In case of ingestion of a toxic substance, please call Poison Control.*

ARNICA comes both in the form of homeopathic pellets and topical creams. I prefer creams since pellets often contain dairy (lactose). Arnica not only targets bruising or minor traumas, but also muscle or joint aches. Do not use it on open injuries.

CAYENNE PEPPER capsules are a proven styptic or antihemorrhagic agent. Open the capsule and apply it externally to a cut to stop bleeding. It burns but it's effective.

CALENDULA OINTMENT acts as a natural antibiotic and provides pain relief for minor cuts and scrapes.

CHAMOMILE is a mild calming agent for general discomfort from illnesses or insomnia. It works great as a poultice on teething gums or to treat pinkeye. To prepare, mix equal parts of ground dried chamomile and slippery elm powder, also a soothing demulcent herb. Mix in enough water and raw honey to create a paste. Apply the paste on the affected area and cover with a gauze for one day. A chamomile tea compress can also help pacify sluggish or nervous digestion. Soak a cloth in warm chamomile tea, and place it directly on the abdomen for relief.

CASTOR OIL can be used as a pack to treat any bodily congestion, menstrual pain, and constipation. Gently warm 2 tablespoons of castor oil to dampen a wool cloth. Lie down, apply the cloth to the abdomen and place a hot water bottle over it for an hour.

EUCALYPTUS is a mild and petroleum-free alternative to conventional respiratory balms. For sinus or lung infections, dilute a 1:3 ratio of eucalyptus oil in coconut oil to apply externally on the chest and bottoms of the feet.

MAGNESIUM CITRATE is a gentle muscle relaxer and laxative. Prepare 2 teaspoons of magnesium powder in hot water before bed for constipation relief in the morning.

BAKING SODA is a quick remedy for severe heartburn and urinary tract infection. Dissolve a ¼ teaspoon in water and drink after an uncomfortable meal or when experiencing urinary tract infection pain. It also stops cold sores from forming when applied as a paste at the first sensation of tingling or redness. Simply mix enough water into baking soda until creamy then apply directly on the cold sore.

NETTLE LEAF prepared as a strong tea provides relief from seasonal allergy and water retention. Combine a 1:4 ratio of herb to hot water and drink throughout the day.

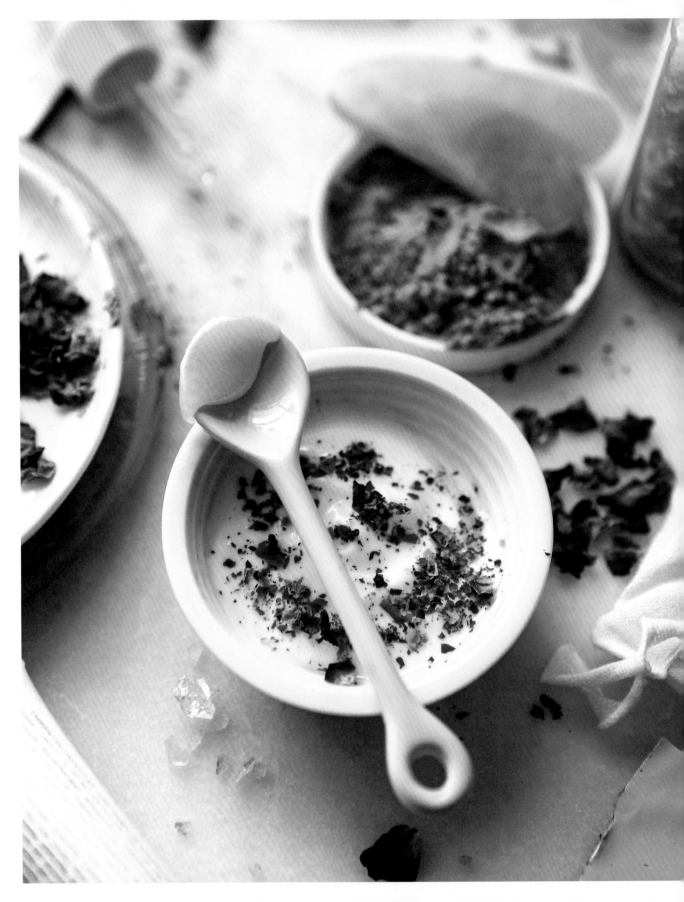

HOLISTIC SKINCARE

Just before my celiac diagnosis, my face broke out in tiny rashes. Having followed a regimen since I was eight years old, I was frustrated with the unexpected outbreak; I would rub my fingers over the rashes in hatred at what my body was doing to me. At the tail-end of puberty, I was expecting to enter a new period of clarity—emotionally and physically—not spiraling back to feeling like an uncomfortable, awkward pubescent.

That's when my aunt offered the most cherished skin advice I have ever received: **BE KIND TO YOUR SKIN**. When we are aggressive toward our skin, whether emotionally hating it or attacking it with harsh products, our skin reacts in kind. Only when we are gentle with our skin will it clear itself of its reactionary tendencies.

CREATE A REGIMEN

Besides the given of opting for plant-derived, non-toxic products, the application of the product is crucial.

1   Begin by lightly spraying your face with **THERMAL SPRING WATER**. It counteracts the drying and acidifying effects of hard water and tap water constituents like chlorine, acting as a softening preparation for the skin to receive the products.

2   Liquify and warm your cleanser in your hands, then use gentle, rapid movements to cleanse your face. The idea here is to cleanse not penetrate the skin. Caress your skin like silk and use effleurage or circular, outward motions by constantly uplifting the skin. Do not neglect the neck, being sure to stroke up against gravity.

3   Rinse with tepid water; any extremes will dry out the skin.

4   Do not use a towel to dry as they often accumulate bacteria; simply wipe off excess water with your hands. Spritz again with thermal water.

5   Spritz **TONER** or **ROSE WATER** on a cotton round to wipe off any remaining dirt. This also makes the skin more receptive to the products that get applied next.

6   Place a drop of your chosen serum on your fingers and gently dab it on your cheeks, forehead, and chin until fully absorbed. Again, treat your skin like silk, ever so delicately.

7   Follow this with facial **GUA SHA** (see Note below). This can be done by gently scraping the face, away from the midline, with a *gua sha* tool. Start from the nose

Continues

out to the ears on both sides; from the center of the eyebrows up to the hairline; above the eyebrows horizontally out towards the temples; from the chin out towards the ears; and from the ears down to the collarbone.

8   Moisturize oily or imbalanced skin using a light serum followed by lotion; use a moisturizer for normal or combination skin; and a serum with a rich cream or oil for dry skin. I recommend **CAMELLIA OIL**, which is the most treasured oil of Japanese geishas. It is rich in oleic acid and vitamins A, B, D, and E; high in Omega 3, 6, and 9; and contains more naturally occurring antioxidants than any other plant-derived oil. To apply, warm the moisturizer on your fingers then apply with uplifting, outward movements to counteract gravity.

9   Perform **PIANOTAGE**, gently tapping the fingers around your face as if playing the piano to increase circulation and hydration. Warm your hands then gently press them on your face.

10   To finish, apply eye cream by dabbing a smudge at the corners of and below the eyes. Dab any excess on the upper lip, an area highly prone to signs of aging. Gently caress the cream around the eyes, up toward the eye sockets, and out in circular motions. Follow this with a sunscreen if it's in the morning.

MAKE THIS

Magical Miel Mask

1 teaspoon **raw honey**

1 teaspoon raw, **grass-fed yogurt**

1 teaspoon **red** or **green clay**

1 drop of **chamomile essential oil**

Spread on clean skin, let dry for 20 minutes, then wash. Apply weekly.

Treat your regimen as bookends to your days, a time to be in higher contact with yourself. Envelop your skin in a silky cocoon dense with indulgent self-care.

NOTE   *Benefits of skin scraping or gua sha include: increase in collagen production, even skin tone, dark circle and puffiness reduction, increased lymphatic drainage and circulation, and pore size reduction.*

ESSENTIAL OILS

Essential oils are natural aromatic compounds extracted from parts of a plant such as its seeds, roots, or flowers. When you peel a grapefruit, for instance, the aromas you experience are the fragrant essential oils contained within the rind. These oils not only provide plants their scent but also imbue them with protective antiviral, antibacterial, antiseptic, and anti-inflammatory properties. Each plant has a delicate ratio of medicinal constituents that provide it with specific benefits. Some common uses are improving immunity, balancing hormones, air purification, detoxification, and creating household or beauty products.

As they are highly concentrated and non-water-soluble phytochemical extractions, essential oil usage requires caution. More is not always better with essential oils as they are immediately absorbed by the skin. Every essential oil has different ratios for dilution and they should be applied accordingly as too much can actually be harmful. Please consult a handbook on essential oils or a trusty website such as www.doterra.com or www.youngliving.com for further information on dilution ratios. Essential oils are concentrated sources of plants, which means not only does one drop contain a potent source of the plant's properties but requires an immense amount of the plant material. Mindful usage is not only beneficial for your body but also for the sustainability of the environment. Also read any precautions or contraindications, such as a medical condition or pregnancy, before using any oil.

Another point of caution is the quality of the essential oil. Although some can be quite expensive, high-quality essential oils are extracted from a great concentration of plants. Unlike inferior-quality oils, they pass third-party testing and are not diluted with carrier oils. Additionally, look for organic options to avoid contaminants such as pesticides.

I recommend using essential oils topically and for diffusing only, as the research behind ingestion of these oils is still limited. Refer to each essential oil's respective dilution ratio for use in a carrier oil, such as fractionated coconut oil, which stays liquid at all temperatures. Aromatherapy, or the diffusing of essential oils, is also beneficial as the oils can enter the bloodstream gently through inhalation. Make sure they're un- or low-heated diffusers as essential oils are very temperature sensitive.

To create a starter kit of essential oils, start with the ones below which are gentle, accessible, and multipurpose.

PEPPERMINT is the essential oil to relieve any neurovascular tension such as headaches, migraines, or overdriven lymphatic system due to a compromised immune system. Applying peppermint oil can even reduce these pains as effectively as 1,000 mg of acetaminophen. Although peppermint is soothing, it also is clarifying by lifting issues such as inability to focus. Dilute it in a carrier oil to use with a roll-on applicator on points of tension such as the temples, nape of the neck, and shoulders.

ROSEMARY stimulates lymph circulation, hair growth, and energetic flow. Add it to your shampoo or hair mask for healthy hair or massage it with a carrier oil after dry brushing to open energetic channels.

TEA TREE or **MALELEUCA** is cleansing for both the household and the skin. Dilute it in white vinegar for an antimicrobial surface cleaner or in a carrier oil to dab it on breakouts.

LAVENDER, the most well-studied essential oil, is one for balance. It aids in the regulation of hormones, emotions, digestion, and neurovascular system to tame headaches or bodily pains. Its sedative effects can relieve menstrual symptoms through aromatherapy in as little as ten minutes.[10] To induce deeper sleep, diffuse it in an air diffuser according to the manufacturer's directions before going to bed.

CITRUS oils such as orange, lemon, and lime act as antiseptics to stimulate the immune system. They are also mood elevators. Take caution when using these photosensitive oils as they increase sensitivity to sunlight and can consequently stain the skin. For an all-purpose cleaner, combine 30 drops of lemon, grapefruit, or orange essential oil with 20 drops of tea tree essential oil. Add 2 cups of distilled white vinegar and 2 cups of water along with a teaspoon of natural dish soap.

FRANKINCENSE is a multipurpose body oil, easing the spiritual, emotional, and physical bodies. It relieves anxiety and anger, strengthens meditation and spiritual connection, and is an anti-pathogenic analgesic to relieve pain while speeding recovery. It also contains sesquiterpenes, which cross the blood-brain barrier to stimulate the limbic system in control of memory and emotions. For a quick pain-relieving ointment, dilute 20 ounces each of frankincense, myrrh, and ginger essential oils in 4 ounces of unrefined coconut oil.

CLARY SAGE is a pain reliever and tames tension, especially caused by hormonal imbalances or menstruation. It contains estrogenic properties to balance hormone levels in the body, such as reducing cramping.[11] Marjoram essential oil also has a similar effect. For a hormone-balancing oil to rub on the abdomen for cramping or pre-menstrual symptom prevention, combine 3 drops of clary sage with 5 drops of lavender in an ounce of a carrier oil, such as fractionated coconut oil or jojoba oil.

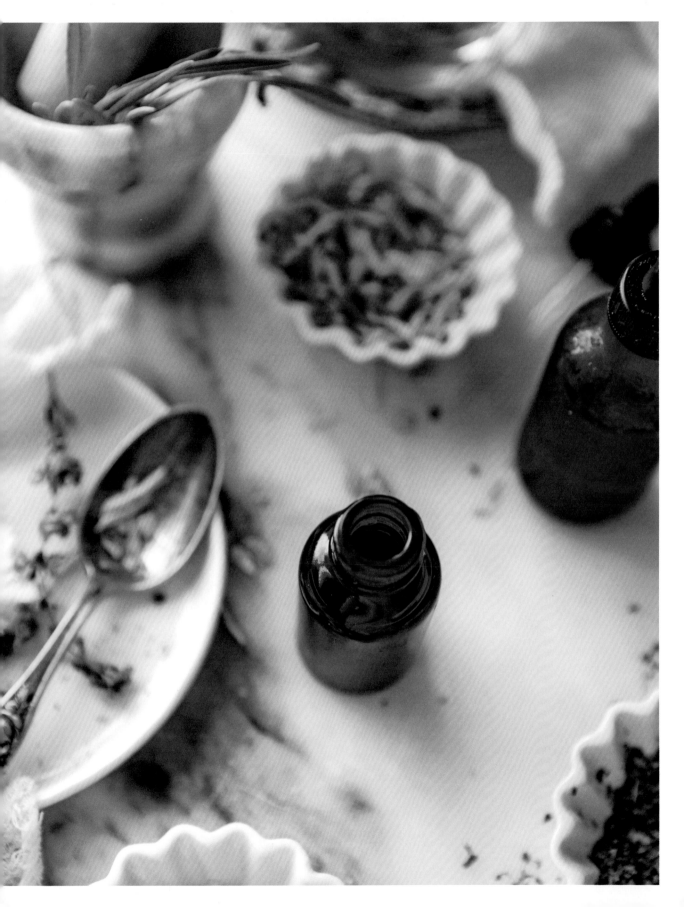

GENTLE CLEANSING
& CLEARING

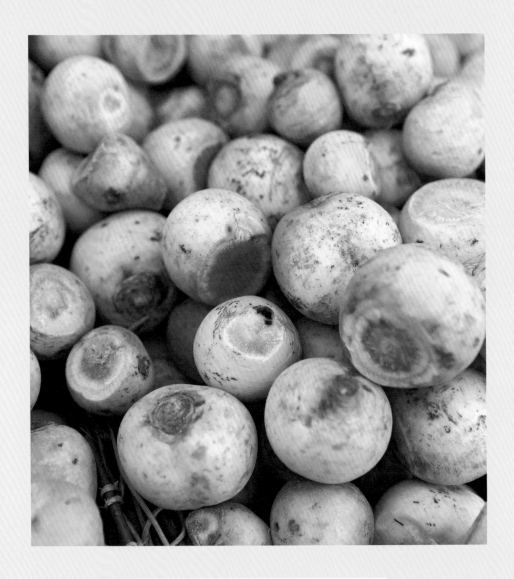

According to Traditional Chinese Medicine (TCM), spring is the best time for detoxification or cleansing our liver function. The cold aggravates the liver, both from the external environment or internal conditions created through nutrition such as eating cold foods. When this happens, the liver becomes clogged, sluggish, or works improperly, causing slow elimination, dry skin, acne, brain fog, fatigue, irritability, accumulation of toxins—both physical and energetic—and cravings. Nourishing the liver during early winter gently grounds the body to make space for us to welcome in the renewal of spring.

KITCHEN

Spices not only heighten the flavor and aromas of a meal, but infuse medicinal qualities that can enhance absorption. Incorporate fresh and dried turmeric, ginger, oregano, mint, thyme, and cinnamon to warm the system. Cinnamon is especially heating and balances out blood sugar levels that can teeter with the seasonal cravings for sweets. Lemons and limes also optimize liver function by alkalizing the body and addressing the liver's preference for pungent or sour tastes. Other sour incorporations include fermented foods such as sauerkraut (page 178), kombucha (page 174), or kvass (a fermented drink made from rye bread), and enzymatic additions such as raw apple cider vinegar.

TURMERIC AND GINGER are energizing and warming yet soothing. Their astringent and bitter properties aid the body in digesting the odd food combinations or indulgences that are a signature of the cold seasons.

TEA OF DANDELION OR BURDOCK ROOT, MARSHMALLOW ROOT, SLIPPERY ELM, and **ASHITABA** are good ways to hydrate during the cleansing season of spring. Dandelion and burdock root are especially detoxifying, acting as a gentle broom for the digestive tract. Marshmallow root and slippery elm are digestive lubricants for proper assimilation of nutrients, movement, and elimination of accumulated toxins. Ashitaba is a supportive addition to build blood when the colder seasons pool it away from our extremities.

RADISHES are called "the little ginseng" in TCM, touted to be the equivalent of "an apple a day." Although radishes are cooling foods, they provide hydration for the body and aid in elimination of waste that can become stagnant in the cold and indulgent seasons. They provide the body with pungency and bitterness for liver function that can be heightened with the inclusion of other foods such as dark leafy greens and fresh herbs.

Increase your intake of **GHEE** and **COCONUT OIL** during the winter. Ghee delivers internal lubrication and eliminates toxins or *ama* from the body. It increases the benefits of herbs tenfold when mixed with raw, unfiltered honey, allowing for a deeper penetration of medicinal effects by acting as a carrier to the cells. Coconut oil's antimicrobial properties and saturated fats curb cravings and optimize energy levels required to cleanse the system.

The ayurvedic digestive tonic of **TRIPHALA** or three fruits—*amalaki*, *bibhitaki*, and *haritaki*—is a potent antioxidant and mild laxative aid for the season. Unlike other cleansing or expectorating agents, it assists the supportive elements already in place and elimination of toxins. If you have a sensitive or already compromised system, take triphala with caution as it can be too drying for some bodies.

Outside of the kitchen, incorporate **DRY BRUSHING** and **ABHYANGA** (page 60), **MAGNESIUM** (page 14), and **TONGUE SCRAPING** (page 53) to stimulate a lymphatic and cleansing flush.

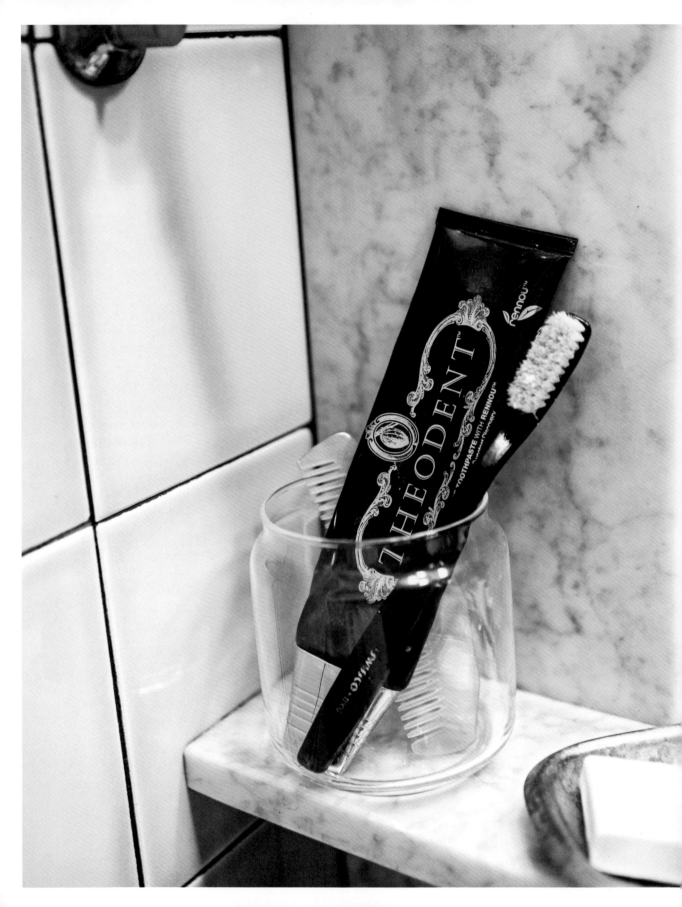

HOLISTIC DENTAL HEALTH

The mouth is a portal to the inner body. The tissue (epithelium) inside the mouth is only one-cell thick and has an absorption rate of over 90 percent.[12] Yet many dental products on the market contain toxic chemicals that make their way into the bloodstream through the mouth's epithelium. These include carcinogenic triclosan, sodium laureth sulfate, and fluoride to name a few, which hinder hormones, immunity, and the microflora balance of the digestive system.

The teeth can instead benefit from the molecular matter found in phytonutrients and botanicals, which also stimulate digestive juices, parathyroid glands, and the hypothalamus. Antibacterial, antiviral essential oils such as **CINNAMON**, **CLOVE**, and **NEEM** not only promote healthy oral ecology but also benefit the rest of the body by being absorbed through the mouth's epithelium.

Opt for an **IONIC TOOTHBRUSH**, which removes plaque from the teeth by repelling it. Ionic toothbrushes temporarily reverse the surface polarity of teeth from negative to positive, repelling positively charged plaque through the negatively charged toothbrush head.

> "The blood that runs through your tooth will run through your toe in one minute."
>
> —TIMOTHY A. KERSTEN, DDS

A **TONGUE CLEANER** is an essential part of your holistic oral regimen. When the tongue is gently scraped, *ama*, or toxic accumulations, is expelled, digestion is stimulated, and bad breath is kept at bay. I recommend stainless steel tongue cleaners as opposed to plastic ones as they are much more sterile and less aggressive. Steel tongue cleaners also deposit silver ions on the tongue, providing additional antimicrobial healing.

Rubbing **RAW, UNTOASTED, UNREFINED SESAME OIL** around your gums and teeth after cleaning the teeth is an excellent addition to keep up oral health as it soothes the gums and prevents plaque.

The teeth and gums can also benefit from a regular rubbing of herbal preparations that are like a form of medicinal food. An **AYURVEDIC MIXTURE** of a teaspoon each of **TRIPHALA**, **NEEM POWDER**, and **LODHRA** provides antioxidants and strengthens the teeth. They can all be found in most Asian markets or online.

Within the ayurvedic tradition, **OIL PULLING** invloves swishing **HEALING OILS** in the mouth to cleanse and detoxify. There are two techniques: one is called *gandusha* and the other is *kavala graha*. The former is when the mouth is completely filled with a prepared fluid without any room to gargle or pull, while the latter is when the mouth is filled halfway so that there is room to gargle. Both approaches are suitable for all constitutions and are equally beneficial when practiced often.

Continues

For **GANDUSHA**, you simply fill your mouth with your chosen oil with no room to gargle to hold for three minutes. Spit into the trash then brush your teeth.

KAVALA GRAHA can be done with different preparations depending on the constitution. Ayurvedic texts recommend that oil pulling is practiced ideally first thing in the morning. Contain one or two tablespoons of the oil in your mouth and rinse and pull the oil through the teeth. Start at five minutes and build up to twenty minutes. Don't be alarmed if this causes the eyes to tear and the nose to run—it's a way for the body to expel toxic accumulations contained in the ears, nose, mouth, and eyes. Also within the ayurvedic tradition, different sections of the tongue are connected to specific organs, and oil pulling allows for their purification.

After pulling, spit in the trash, rinse the mouth with water, and brush the teeth. Avoid spitting it in the sink as the formulation now contains harmful toxins that would then contaminate the water sources or cause drain blockages. These oral cleansing techniques will relieve dental issues like plaque buildup and sensitive gums, but also non-dental issues such as dry skin, impaired vision, and sinus congestion.

Another type of **KAVALA GRAHA** calls for filling the mouth halfway with the appropriate preparation below and then gargled. Bring the preparations to a boil and then simmer for five minutes. The oil for the vata preparation should be added after the simmer. Both the vata and kapha formulations should be used warm while the pitta one should be cooled down. Once the preparation is ready, hold it in your mouth for a minute, swish it around, then spit it in the trash. Note that for kapha and pitta constitutions, oil should be avoided.

Mix 1 cup of water with the dosha: For **VATA**, mix with 3 teaspoons of **RAW, UNTOASTED, UNREFINED SESAME OIL** and a ½ teaspoon of **CUMIN SEEDS**. For **KAPHA** constitution, mix with 1 teaspoon of **FENNEL SEEDS**. For **PITTA**, mix with a ½ teaspoon of fresh **GINGER** and a teaspoon of **RAW HONEY**.

Kavala graha by *Dosha*

In ayurvedic medicine, every body has a specific constitution or *prakriti* that affects their dental health. The constitution of an individual determines his or her *dosha*, or mind-body type: *vata, pitta,* and *kapha*. Dental and overall wellness recommendations correlate to the dominance of one of these doshas. To determine yours, simply take a comprehensive online test such as one by Banyan Botanicals (banyanbotanicals.com).

For **vata** constitutions, mix 2 tablespoons of raw, **untoasted, unrefined sesame oil** with either ⅛ teaspoon of **licorice powder** or **high-quality salt**, which aid in the healing of vata imbalances that can manifest in receding or sensitive gums.

Kapha constitutions will benefit from 2 tablespoons of **ghee** prepared with additions such as a drop of **eucalyptus** or **neem oil**, which guard against infections and dryness to which kapha constitutions are susceptible.

Bitter fluids are the most beneficial for **pitta** constitutions, so 2 tablespoons of **ghee** mixed with ½ teaspoon of **neem** or *guduchi* powder will aid in the healing of pitta problems such as bleeding gums, canker sores, and possible white coating of the tongue due to yeast overgrowth.

RESTORATION HAIRCARE

Considering the frequency with which we wash ourselves, it is crucial to also recognize the ingredients that we consequently expose ourselves to. When we opt for conventional and, yes, often cheaper alternatives, we also opt to wash ourselves with toxins and endocrine disruptors. Repeated exposure to these industrial toxins can eventually lead to hormonal irregularities.

LATHER

More than 90 percent of shampoos contain variations of sulfates or polyethylene glycol (PEG) despite clinical studies showing them to not only irritate the skin but disrupt hormones. Generic emulsifiers like PEG also contain carcinogens such as 1,4-dioxane. Alternatives like **COCO PROTEINS** and **YUCCA ROOT** provide a luxurious lather without the effects of toxic surfactants. Instead, they nourish your hair with a nutrient-dense profile of sugars, proteins, and fatty acids.

SCENT

Most people mistakenly believe that switching to a natural shampoo would mean stepping out of the shower with their hair wafting the scents of a head shop or nothing at all. Quite the contrary! **ESSENTIAL OILS** are concentrated plant extracts with potent scents—their fragrance often lasts longer than the artificial ones found in conventional shampoos. They also allow you to avoid the detrimental effects synthetic fragrances have on our bodies. The FDA does not regulate components of substances labeled "fragrance," leading many manufacturers to stockpile toxic chemicals. Avoid synthetic fragrances and their unknown components.

STRENGTH

Retinyl acetate, a form of vitamin A, is often added to conventional strengthening shampoos and conditioners. Although vitamin A found organically in foods such as dark leafy greens is a powerful way to feed your hair, retinyl acetate in haircare leads instead to overexposure to this vitamin. Vitamin A overexposure can cause endocrinological and reproductive issues, as well as weaker, brittle hair. Wheat and soy proteins are overprocessed with toxins and can also lead to itchy or dry scalp. Opt instead for **OAT STRAW** if not diagnosed with celiac or **HORSETAIL**, both of which rebuild the hair shaft through compounds like silica and proteins.

Continues

MOISTURE

Glycerin is another overprocessed substance that is often combined with toxic chemicals. Although it does coat the hair, it can lead to a heavy build up and weigh hair down. Ingredients like **ALOE VERA**, **MARSHMALLOW**, and **YUCCA** are moisturizing botanicals that also promote hair growth, softness, and manageability.

FEED THE FOUNDATION

Healthy hair cannot grow out of a malnourished body. Supplementing with and regularly consuming healthy fats such as coconut oil, high-quality olive oil, grass-fed ghee, and wild-caught seafood is essential. Snacking on **RAW, SPROUTED NUTS AND SEEDS** also feeds hair—think chia seeds, walnuts, almonds, and macadamia nuts. **SPROUTED PUMPKIN SEED MILK** is an easily assimilated milk to support hair growth with an abundant source of zinc, sulfur, and vitamin A. Switch your snacks to **COCONUT BUTTER** for a quick source of saturated fat that supports healthy hormone levels and supports healthy strands.

Adequate consumption of **HIGH-QUALITY PROTEIN**—pasture-raised meats and wild-caught seafood—is necessary for healthy hair growth since hair is composed of protein (keratin). Balance the high level of tryptophan in muscle meat by supplementing with bone broth for easily assimilated protein.

For our bodies to process any proteins, however, we first need a **STRONG DIGESTIVE SYSTEM** and **BALANCED STOMACH ACID** capable of breaking down amino acids. This requires adequate levels of digestive enzymes. A high-functioning digestive system supports efficient metabolism and hormone production, which stimulates hair growth. If you suspect indigestion, speak with your health care practitioner about supporting your diet with high-quality digestive enzymes.

Ayurvedic Hair Mask

3 heaping spoonfuls of **unrefined sesame seed oil** or **raw organic coconut oil**

1 drop of **rosemary essential oil**

1 heaping spoonful of **raw honey**

1 tablespoon of **amla powder**

Add the sesame seed or coconut oil, along with the rosemary essential oil, to a small glass container or jar. Place the container in a pot and add water until level with the oil. Turn stove to medium heat and leave until the jar is warm to the touch. Carefully remove from heat and combine the oil with the honey and amla powder. Mix well and apply to hair, beginning by massaging it into the scalp and following to the ends of the hair. Keep the mask on for at least half an hour to up to an hour. Rinse well with lukewarm water, follow with shampoo and conditioner, and finish off with cold water to seal the moisture into the hair.

Our SCALP *has*

more than
200
Blood Vessels

650
Sweat Glands

1K
Nerve Endings

200K
Hair Follicles

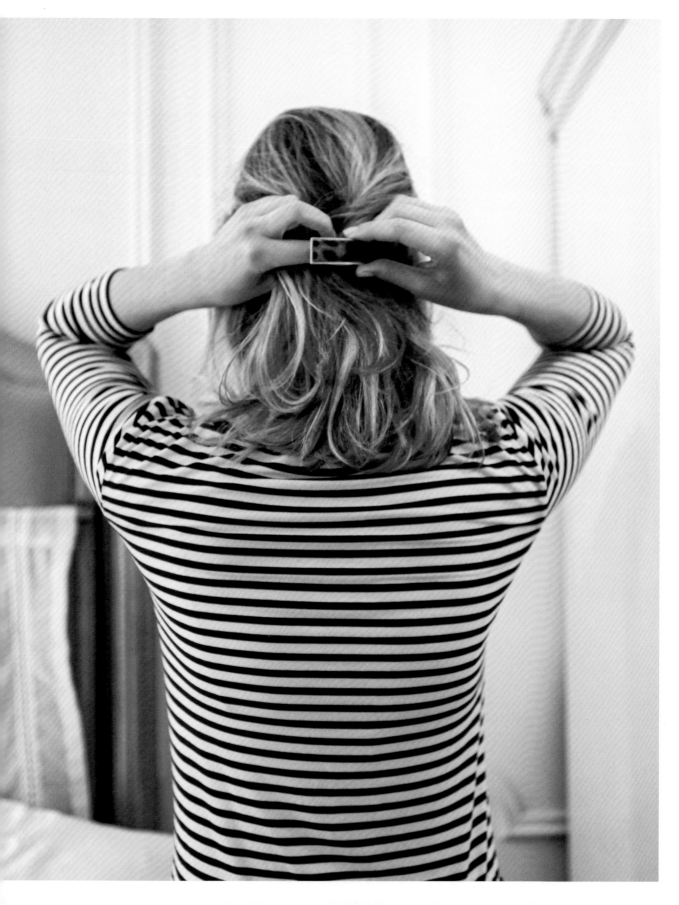

RECOVERING FROM EXERCISE

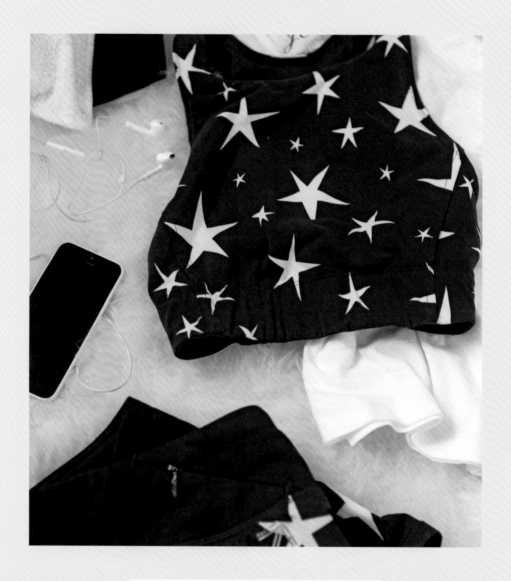

When training or exercising, the body operates in the sympathetic nervous system, dictating action by using adenosine triphosphate (ATP) for fuel. On the other hand, the parasympathetic nervous system uses fat as fuel and is activated during rest. Below are measures I once took to restore my body from illness. Now I take them to help aid athletic recovery and build endurance. Whether it's yoga or long distance running, incorporate these into your pre- and post-workout regimen for optimal performance.

Rest yourself physically and mentally by **MEDITATING** (page 25), oxygenating with **BREATHWORK** to regenerate tissues (page 21), and **SELF-MASSAGE** (page 60). **AROMATHERAPY** with essential oils (page 47) before bed will further stimulate restoration during sleep.

Some stress, however, is beneficial. Exercise in itself is a stressor to the body. With proper recovery, the body adapts to this stress. Without recovery, exercise can cause degeneration, illness, and early aging. When we equip our body with the proper sources of renewal, the breakdown of stress will result in strengthening.

When the body is not adequately nourished following exercise, it self-medicates by generating cravings for nutrients, such as for chocolate when lacking in magnesium and carbohydrates. Complement your training with a **NUTRIENT-DENSE, WHOLE FOOD DIET** consisting of high quality protein from grass-fed meats, wild-caught seafood, or nuts and seeds such as hemp; vegetables; complex grain-free carbohydrates; and essential fatty acids.

Keep your protein-to-carbohydrate ratio 1:1 or 1:2 for **ENDURANCE TRAINING**. For carbohydrates, opt for **ROOT VEGETABLES** such as roasted carrots, sweet potatoes, and winter squashes; **LOW-GLYCEMIC FRUITS** such as berries, avocado, and green apples. Eating carbohydrates post-training will aid in glycogen storage and thus muscle repair.

MAKE THIS

Pre-workout Tonic

Blend **½ teaspoon** each of **cordyceps powder** and **cinnamon**, **1 tablespoon** of **maca powder**, **1 teaspoon** of **coconut oil** or **ghee**, and **stevia** to taste in a hot but not boiling **cup** of **nut milk**.

Post-workout Tonic

Blend **½ teaspoon** of **reishi**, **¼ teaspoon** of **mesquite**, **½** a **banana** or **1 date**, and **½** an **avocado** with **1 cup** of **nut milk**.

Opt for **HIGH-ALKALINE** and **HIGH-CHLOROPHYLL VEGETABLES**, such as dark greens; seaweeds such as chlorella; fresh herbs like cilantro; and nutrient-dense sprouts. Chlorophyll aids in reducing oxidation from stress, repairs cells with nucleic acids, and stabilizes insulin levels.

Include **PREBIOTIC FOODS** as well, such as raw garlic and onion or bananas; the latter also supplies electrolytes and carbohydrates for muscle repair.

Supplement this diet with **B VITAMINS, OMEGA-3 OILS**, and **ADAPTOGENS** for increased performance. B vitamins are responsible for efficiently utilizing carbohydrates and fats for energy production as well as blood oxygenation. Add liposomal or ash-derived vitamin B complex for endurance. Take liposomal vitamin C post-training with L-glutamine, which work synergistically to restore glycogen levels and collagen production for muscle repair. Add adaptogens to allow your body to adapt to the stress of exercise.

MASSAGE

A physical body at ease allows for energetic movement and space for our emotional bodies to be at ease, too. Before you perform the following massages, begin with the exercise on page 99 to communicate with your esoteric body. This is your energetic field or the immediate contact that aligns your emotional associations in higher bodies with your physical one.

LYMPHATIC DRAINAGE and *ABHYANGA* are massage practices of conscious ritual, infusing intention behind every move. Through body awareness, these daily exercises become a means to transform mundane, repetitive acts into a time for listening to our own constitution, unimpeded by any external forces.

Lymphatic drainage begins with dry skin brushing or *GARSHANA*, an ancient practice of sweeping the body gently with raw silk or a natural vegetable brush to remove dead skin and stimulate the lymphatic system. This reinvigorates the nervous system through nerve and systemic organ stimulation; detoxifies fat tissues that store accumulated toxins; and allows the lymph canals to flush toxic metabolic wastes via the colon. It also tightens the skin by rejuvenating blood flow, increases collagen production for cell renewal, and opens up the pores for better moisture absorption.

Dry skin brushing consequently makes the following practice of **ABHYANGA**, the ayurvedic practice of self-oil-massage, more beneficial. Massaging oil into stimulated, open pores provides increased hydration and allows moisture to penetrate deeper into the cells. Lubricating the body with oil also taps into the *ojas* or life force circulating deep within the skin tissue, increasing longevity,

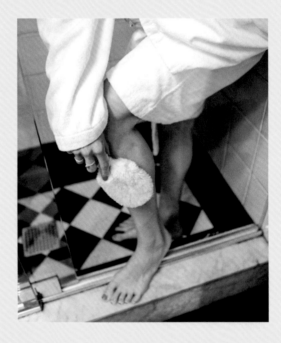

joint mobility, and digestion. It is a humbling experience to feel the increased energy flow permeating from our own hands. A dear friend once pointed out to me that the Sanskrit word *sneha* can be translated as both "oil" and "love," unveiling the self-love that this oiling ritual generates.

Please abstain from this practice if you are menstruating, have mass-like inflammation, are acutely ill or recovering, pregnant, or have a thick, white coating on your tongue that is indicative of high levels of *ama*.

GARSHANA (DRY BRUSHING)

Dry brushing should be performed on dry skin, once per day, and ideally first thing in the morning as it's an energizing practice. The strokes should be long, sweeping, and gentle, moving in the direction of the heart. Begin from the feet with long strokes upwards along the legs. Continue on to the torso with upward strokes in the area below the belly button and for the buttocks, and downward strokes from the chin down to the belly button. Follow with upward strokes for both arms. Use upwards strokes for the back until the back of the neck, where downwards strokes finish the body brushing.

NOTE *Avoid dry brushing on your face, on damaged skin, or during your menstrual cycle.*

ABHYANGA MASSAGE

1 Abhyanga can range anywhere from five to sixty minutes, anytime of day. Begin by lightly warming a small glass bowl of oil in hot water and lay a towel down in a comfortable area. Undress completely.

2 Apply the warm oil starting at the feet, massaging each toe. Use slow, upward, gentle strokes on the limbs and circular ones around the joints.

3 Move up to the legs with long, gentle strokes toward the knees, switch to massaging circularly around the joint, then in upward strokes toward the hips. Repeat for each leg.

4 Move from the lower back to the outer hips with gentle strokes then up toward the back.

5 Massage the belly in clockwise circles from the navel to stimulate digestion.

6 Move up to the chest and massage towards the clavicles, then move towards the arms, hands, and each finger.

7 Finish with the neck, face, and scalp by massaging the face with outward strokes. Massage the ears and give your scalp a gentle rub. Let the oil soak in if you have the time, preferably meditating for ten minutes.

HEALING SALVES FOR BURNS, SCARS, & SCRAPES

As a precaution, do not ice your burns. Drastically cold temperatures shock skin tissue and can damage it further than it already has been by restricting blood flow. Simply run the burnt area under cool water or keep it under cool water for around twenty minutes before applying the treatments below.

The astringent, cooling, and tissue-regenerative properties of **ALOE VERA** soothe burns while speeding up the recovery process. If you're ideally using an actual aloe plant, pluck off a leaf then slit it lengthwise. Scoop out the gel inside and apply it directly onto the burn.

Simply cut a thin slice of **RAW POTATO,** which is full of soothing enzymes, starch, and vitamin C to promote recovery and prevent blisters. Apply a cool, thin slice on affected area for twenty minutes.

Not only does **RAW HONEY** work as an antiseptic in protecting your burn from getting infected, the active enzymes in raw, unheated, and unfiltered honey aid in removing the dead skin cells and regenerating healthy skin tissue.

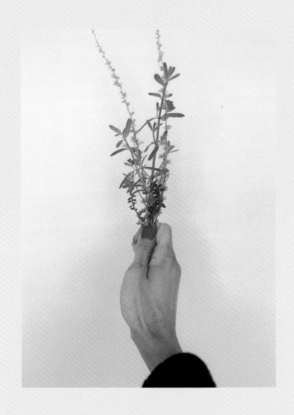

CALENDULA is one of the most potent plants for healing any skin condition, from acne scars to wounds. You can liberally apply calendula cream on the affected area for recovery support.

RAW MILK is one of the most effective pain relievers as a compress. The fat, protein, and enzymes in raw milk soothe the burn and provide hydration. Make a paste with the milk and baking soda, apply on the affected area, and cover with a breathable light cotton gauze.

APPLE CIDER VINEGAR is another remedy full of enzymes that dissolve dead skin cells and prevent infection. Make sure it's diluted in water as straight apple cider vinegar may further irritate tender skin.

COOL TEA such as green or black variety is one of the most effective remedies for treating sunburned and itchy skin. Boil a combination of 2 tablespoons each of mint, green, and plantain leaf tea. Let cool, then apply the tea with a soaked cotton towel.

Burnt skin is dehydrated skin. Proper hydration is essential with mineralizing sea salts and rehydrating herbal teas. Rather than chugging cups of water, hack into your body's hydration regulation with a 2-ounce shot of ALOE VERA JUICE and HERBAL TEAS. Aloe vera lubricates our insides while gynostemma, raspberry leaf, and rooibos teas provide deeper levels of moisture into the tissues than drinking pure water does.

HELICHRYSUM and LAVENDER ESSENTIAL OILS, diluted either in 2 ounces of water to be used as a spray or in fractionated coconut oil, can heal scars that have already manifested. Tea tree oil with diluted witch hazel is also effective in preventing infection of burns and pain.

Massaging oils onto burns and scars is one of the best ways to recirculate the blood and promote energy flow for the reconstruction of new tissue once the burn itself has healed and is no longer tender. CARROT SEED, ROSEHIP, and OLIVE OILS are deeply healing options for healing scars. COCONUT OIL is a cooling option for burns and its lauric acid content aids in burn wound contraction to lessen the chance of scarring.

VITAMIN C promotes wound healing and diminishes scars by increasing collagen production, which is the building block for repairing and generating new skin. Liposomal vitamin C is a bioavailable version of this antioxidant that is transferred straight into the bloodstream to be directed into our cellular tissues that need regenerative support. VITAMIN E is an antioxidant—dabbing up to 1,000 mg daily straight on the skin or consuming more olive-oil-rich vitamin E will speed up the process of healing.

Traditional ancestral diets included plenty of dietary sources of gelatin and collagen with regular consumption of bone broth, calves foot jelly, and organ meats. Collagen hydrolysate and gelatin are composed of 35 percent glycine and 21 percent proline and hydroxyproline, which is balancing for the hormones, skin tissue, the gut, and the musculoskeletal structure. Supplement your diet with bone broth or purchase collagen and gelatin powder from grass-fed animals if your diet permits it. NETTLE LEAF is a great plant-based alternative for mineralizing and strengthening the musculoskeletal structure as well. You can drink a few cups of it as a tea.

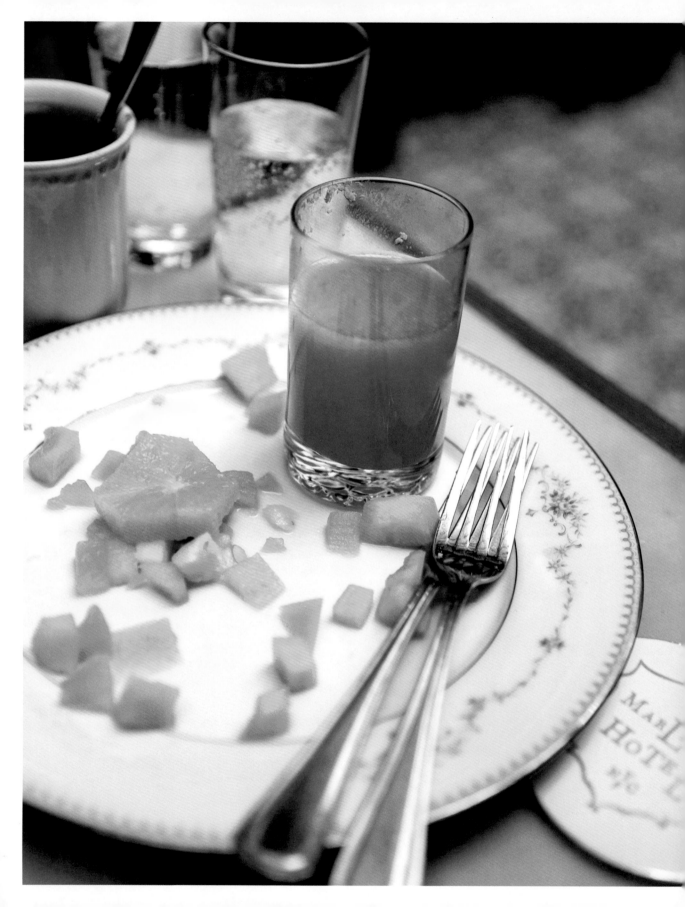

MINDFUL EATING

Eating is a practice, honed over time through emotional and physical associations. When we rush through our meals, we repeat a mindless cycle of immediate hunger gratification, raising another forkful before we've swallowed the last. Rather, eating should be a time when we can slow down to savor and receive the nourishment contained in each bite. It's not necessarily a meditation—we're not sitting down as Buddha before our plates—but rather a sitting in the presence of your meal; not a time to float in other thoughts or in the microcosm of social media.

For some of us, mindful eating is an opportunity to relearn that we are vessels made to receive nourishment. When we sit at the table, we must empty ourselves of what we're full of emotionally so that we can receive what we are given physically. If you are emotionally full, release your emotions before you eat. If you are emotionally empty or numb, don't view your meal as a mode of feeling or medication.

MEAL TIME MEDITATION

Allow your mealtime to extend beyond the sensations of the taste buds and connect to your entire body. Just as Yogi Bhajan advised in a lecture to touch the body and essentially bless it before a meal, you can develop a practice similar to the following:

Hold your shoulders and feel their strength. Touch your knees and recall where they've taken you and where they will carry you next. Place your hand over your heart as a sign of self-empathy for all that you've faced and are facing. Ask that this meal will keep your heart from habitual mindless reactions. Touch your forehead as a reminder to simultaneously feel and think through your meal. Eating is a language to reconnect the words spoken by your mind, body, and spirit. Break your food down, build yourself up.

ZERO-WASTE LIVING

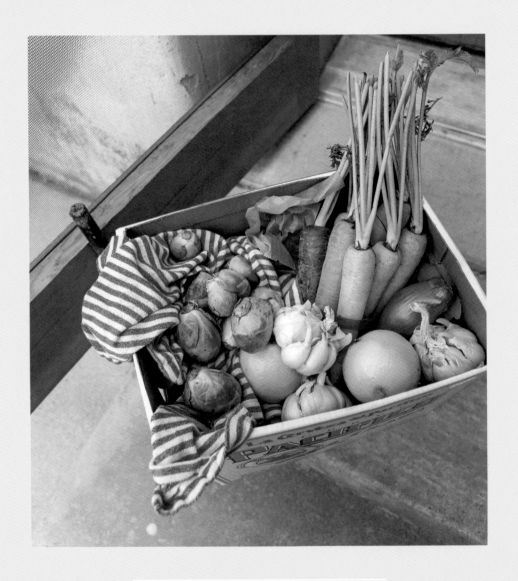

Before embarking on reducing physical and mental trash in our lives, we must notice and acknowledge its presence. The accumulation of trash itself manifests in the mind, as well, since any sort of "clutter," even if stored away, will occupy mental space.

First, observe. Think of why you want to reduce trash and what you are currently doing that is producing more of it. This will create a starting point to focus on. What kind of trash are you mostly producing—is it food containers or un-recyclables from your online shopping deliveries? Why do you want to reduce your waste—is it for environmental impact, minimalism, or a tight budget?

Pat yourself on the back for your responses. It's important to not embark on your journey feeling overwhelmed or critical about your current lifestyle. You've already made a highly aware and impactful decision for yourself and all that is larger than you by beginning a reduced-waste lifestyle.

Next, take the time to energetically clear your physical space. Pick and clear your path with botanicals, such as burning a white sage stick, palo santo, or sweetgrass. You could say a simple internal prayer as you walk around the room wafting the smoke, asking that this physical clearing manifests into a clearing of your mind.

Once you have cleansed the air, prepare to transition to a reduced-waste lifestyle by disposing of your unnecessary items. Identify your daily staples—are there green alternatives? This can be anything from plastic storage containers—even the BPA-free ones—to paper towels. Anything plastic still contains endocrine-disrupting chemicals, such as an equally toxic replacement of BPS (Bisphenol S) and phthalates.[13] Choose cotton towels, glass jars, stainless steel flatware, wood, porcelain, and ceramic instead. Donate or recycle old plastic storage containers and utensils. Use sustainable alternatives for storing leftovers at home or to-go cups at coffee shops. Most recyclables do not make it to the recycling plant and even when they do, there's a limit to how many times they can be recycled.

Let go of items that are no longer used. Most can be donated to Goodwill or sold at a consignment store.

TRY THIS

Zero-Waste

Here are a few simple swaps for your new zero-waste lifestyle:

- **Organic cotton bags** instead of plastic bags for produce
- **Reusable cotton tote bag** instead of disposable plastic grocery bags
- **Stainless steel bottle** instead of plastic bottles
- **Wooden** or **marble cutting board** instead of plastic ones
- **Wooden to-go ware** instead of plastic utensils
- **Stainless steel** and **glass food containers** instead of plastic
- **Cast iron** or **stainless steel** instead of nonstick cookware
- **Cotton towels** instead of paper ones

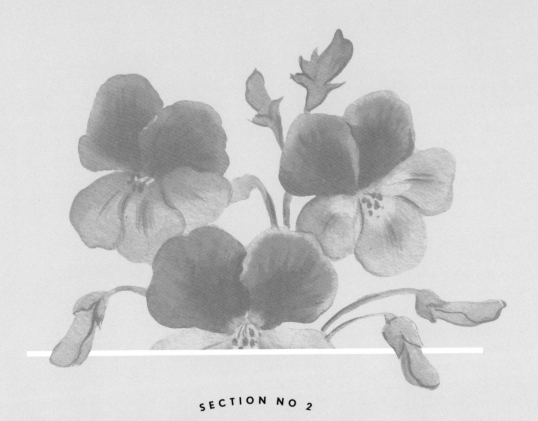

SPIRITUAL SMACK

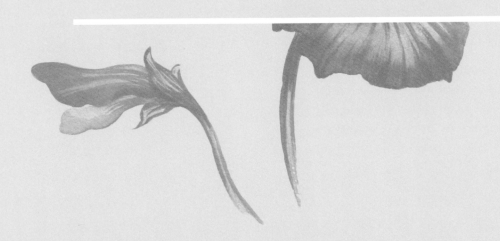

SHORTLY AFTER I *began* MY BLOG,

I started working at the Environmental Working Group (EWG). I would take an hour-plus trip on the DC Metro, which was often over-packed, under construction, or delayed for half an hour. I'd arrive to work earlier than anyone and often be one of the last to leave.

Consequently, I had very minimal time to dedicate to my blog. Coming home at eight at night, I found more comfort in spreading my limbs out on the sofa than locating words for another post. Yet I didn't experience the restoration I was seeking, a solace of my own. This paradox constricted my energy until I had an epiphany riding on the Metro, and I began writing . . . on my iPhone's Reminders app. This started to become a regular occurrence on the Metro, while walking on the street, or in a daze. I even began writing my blog posts while in transit. I had come to surrender my assumptions—that to write, we have to be in a certain mood or place; to achieve a goal, we must have a structured and paved path; and for all, a foreseeable set time.

This section is a compilation of brief visions that lead to lingering, permeating awakenings. It's of revelations that humorously arise while staring at an undone manicure; of sights on the streets that ring of unexpected calls to memories, reminding us of the delicacies of life; of whispers in the dark; and of realizations that smack like a bizarre summer breeze. It's a photojournalistic rumination to guide you into a heightened sense of awareness of the visions both within and around you.

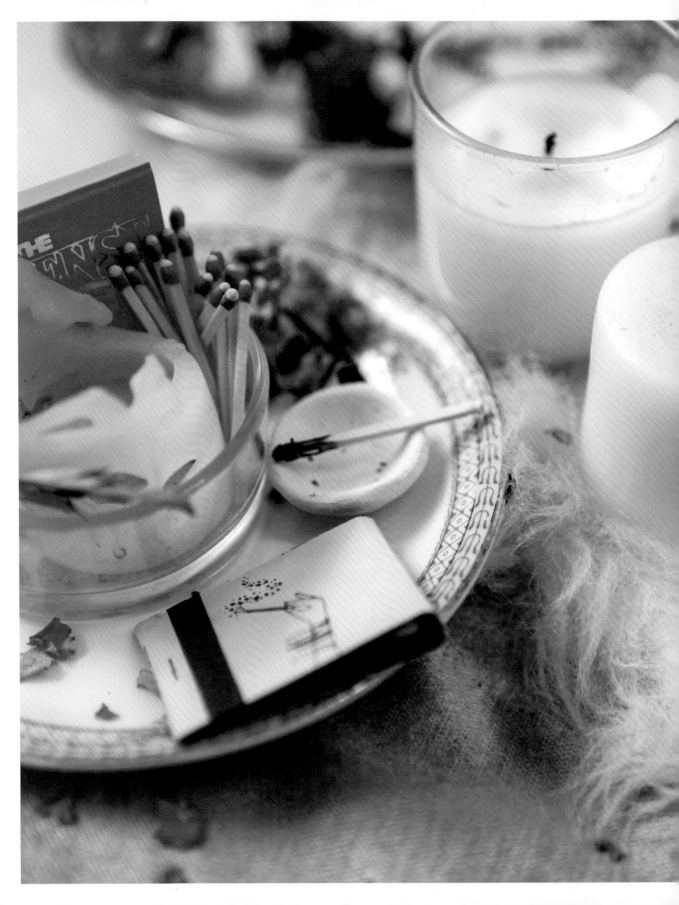

SOFTENING THE SENSES

Amidst increased tension and rush within our days, many of us hastily walk around with furrowed brows, tight lips, and clenched hands. Our bodies become host to the layers of strain in our minds. This not only takes an individual, physical toll, but also a collective one, affecting and creating boundaries against the people in our lives.

How, then, can we soften our senses to open these boundaries? Take the time to refine your relationship with yourself by noticing your habitual mental and physical inclinations. Do you hold your tongue instead of speaking honestly? Do your shoulders cave in when facing your work? How you physically and mentally approach life is how it will approach you in return. Sunken shoulders reflectively submerge our energy—straighten them into a welcoming state of expansion. Choose your words wisely yet tenderly so they may not only extend honesty and knowledge but amplify a curiosity for others to seek that within themselves.

Always return to yourself. Allow the time to grant your body the silence through which it can navigate the freedom to release the tension stored in the crevices of your mind and interactions. Unfurl your brows and soften your gaze. Find room within yourself to open a space of sacredness around you and those with whom you interact with. Lighten the corners of your mouth so that you can release your smile. Heighten your senses to unearth deeper receptivity toward yourself and others.

And please, let yourself truly listen. When you're listening to another and have an immediate response, instead allow their words to settle within you. Then listen to how your response resonates within your body so you can sense how it might resonate with others. Similarly, when you listen to others react to your story or behavior, pause and process them without the knee-jerk need for an immediate response. Consider how your words are heard and absorbed by others, so you may become a voice for not only yourself but those who have been quieted down against their will.

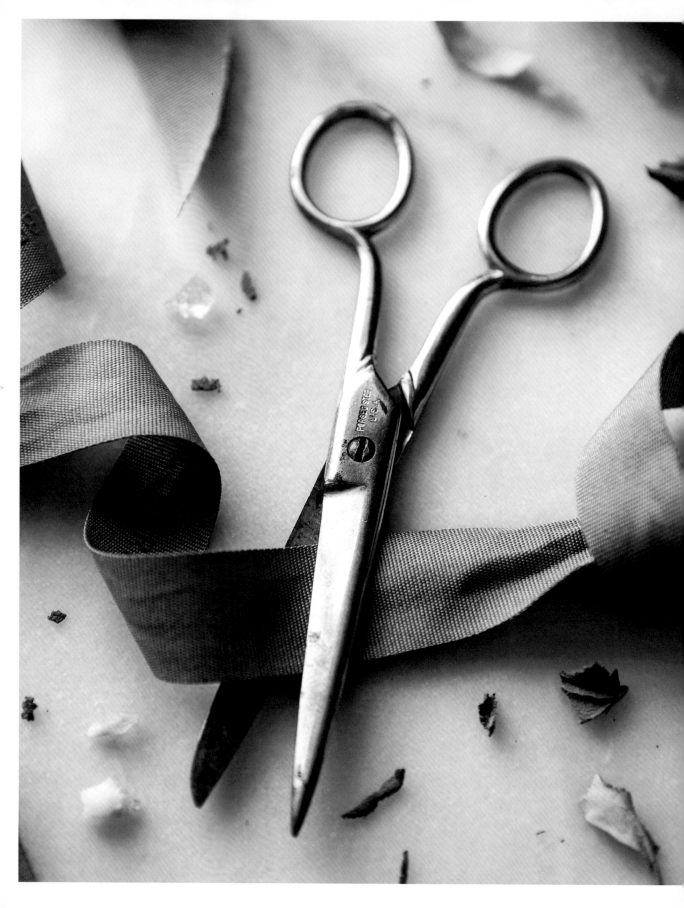

CORD CUTTING

A ceremonial meditation to dissolve draining negative connections to recharge your energy and create abundant opportunities.

Whenever we make a connection with someone, especially romantically, we create energetic or **ETHE-RIC CORDS.** These invisible cords of energy connect the person—a romantic partner, co-worker, friend, or family—to that of our own energetic field. Through our interactions, thoughts, emotions, and mutterings, the activated cords are further strengthened.

Doreen Virtue describes etheric cords as ones that "act like hoses, with energy directed back and forth between both people." These cords are a high-frequency communication tunnel in which we share, transmit, and transmute our energy. It's a telepathic dispatch of our thoughts and emotions.

When these cords are bound in a healthy relationship, they create a source of vibrant energy that elevates our own resources, as in the jolt of energy we get when a loved one contacts us during an afternoon slump.

In an unhealthy etheric connection, the cords bind and drag us down to where we lose control and feel sapped of energy. This is often why we get tired from speaking to, being in the presence of, or even merely thinking about someone we dislike, or about whom we have obsessive, grieving, or fearful thoughts.

We forge etheric cords daily, and it's likely that you intuitively know who feeds your energy and who steals it from you. If you feel your energy is exhausted by someone or you would like to move toward a path of releasing negative patterns or addictions, this cord-cutting ritual is a tool to incorporate into your healing journey.

As a precaution: when we sever and release etheric cords that no longer serve us, the other person will often feel it. Although they will not know the source of this feeling or what it is, they will sense an inexplicable void in you and your energy. They might call, text, or email you. This happens to me more often than not when I practice the cord-cutting ritual. This can pull you into a black hole and back into their negative energetic exchange, especially when it's a romantic partner you're still attracted to but who does not serve you. Do another round of the meditation if necessary until you feel a complete release of their attachments.

THE CORD-CUTTING MEDITATION

Find a space where it's quiet and you feel at ease—this can be in your bedroom, living room, by a spiritual altar, or even in a relaxing bath.

Although it's not necessary, I like to smudge the space with sage or palo santo to clear any negative energies that might affect my meditation.

Take a comfortable seat and gently close your eyes, calling upon whatever universal guide you would like to assist you—G-d, angels, spiritual leaders, your inner guide, et cetera.

Continues

Repeat the following mantra or prayer from Tanaaz Chubb to your spiritual guide, asking for their assistance in releasing this etheric cord that no longer serves you: *"Dear Spirit Guide(s), I call upon you to help me heal, let go, and cut any etheric cords that are no longer serving my higher purpose. I ask that all cords attached to me that are not aligned with love, light, and positive attention be released. Help me to release them and surround me with a healing light to protect me from future attachments. Thank you."*

Now visualize the person from whom you would like to detach cords, standing or sitting in front of you. Feel the strength of the cord tying you to the person and how they drain your energy but do not judge him or her. Simply feel their effect on your energetic field and sense of self.

Begin to visualize the cord dissolving. I find repeating the prayer multiple times assists me in this process of the meditation. You will know if the ritual has worked when you feel lighter. When you feel at ease, charge yourself and your field by imagining a protective shield of white, healing light tipped in gold blanketing you.

Gently open your eyes when you're ready and smudge your surroundings again, take a warm bath, drink water, and replenish your renewed self.

LUNAR MANIFESTATION

The cycles of the moon reveal the innate power of ritual. It is through the structure of ritual that we find meaning so we can ease into our days with a sense of connection. Cultivating awareness of lunar cycles is a reminder of the cyclical nature of life, allowing us to envision new beginnings, plant seeds of intention, and evolve through change.

Just like a seed grows in phases, so can an idea in attunement with lunar cycles. An idea is also a seed, an intangible, energetic one. It can be planted at the beginning of the lunar calendar, with the New Moon marking the beginning of the cycle and the Full Moon ending in release. The seeds of intention are planted during the former to come into fruition during the latter.

The Moon goes through eight phases in every thirty days: New Moon, Crescent Moon, First Quarter Moon, Gibbous Moon, Full Moon, Disseminating Moon, Third Quarter Moon, and the Balsamic Moon. The days for each phase will vary every month, so check a lunar calendar.

THE NEW MOON is for setting goals, challenges, and to envision new experiences. It's the time to tune into what you have now in your hands so you may see clearly what you want to manifest. Write these desires down on a dated sheet of paper with the following statement: "I accept these things or something better into my life now for the highest good and the highest good of all concerned in the perfect time and way."[1]

The last part is crucial as our desires can manifest in unintentionally negative ways, such as a large sum of money as a result of an accident. It also allows the Universe to create not only what will serve all but also serve you "something better" than what might be beyond your imagination. Write your statements in the affirmative "I am" rather than pleading with words like "need" or "want." When your manifestation list is complete, tuck it under crystals to charge under the lunar light and then tuck it away into a safe place in the morning until the next Full Moon.

THE CRESCENT MOON is a period of sprouting, memory, and movement. This is the time to attune your intentions to what you'd like to manifest through your list. Manifestation is not a magical game of sit and wait. You are a co-creator with the Universe. What are *you* going to be working on to realize these desires? The manifestation list is the target, but you must pick up your bow and arrow.

THE FIRST QUARTER MOON is the phase of discomfort, change, or resistance. It's the time to muster the energy to actualize your manifestation list or face what is blocking you from receiving them.

Continues

THE GIBBOUS MOON marks the three days preceding the Full Moon. In anticipation of manifested desires, it's a time to create a balanced structure to welcome in fulfilment. As you meditate, visualize the realization of your list.

THE FULL MOON is a time of gratitude for the abundance, wisdom, and blessings that are currently in your life. Bury your manifestation list in acknowledgement of your growth. Write down a new list of what you'd like to release from your life to make space for your desires. Place the list under a crystal in lunar light.

THE DISSEMINATING MOON allows for release and circulation. It's a time to sow seeds of transformative growth. Quietly meditate through your memory to release harmful, energy-draining thoughts and experiences to reprogram yourself like a computer.

THE THIRD QUARTER MOON is a time for maturation and release of habitual patterns or limitations. If such repeating circumstances or attitudes surface, use the support of this moon to face them.

THE BALSAMIC MOON marks the 72 hours preceding the New Moon, cradling our renewed selves like a newborn. Burn your last list as a sign of rebirth and realization, then light a candle in meditation to symbolize the light that comes from the ashes of release.

U - NIVERSE

Is the world coming *at* you or *from* you? How you arrange your mind determines the arrangement of your life. You carve the pillars in the architecture of your life with your thoughts. You're under constant construction, for higher ground. The early-twentieth-century mystic George Gurdjieff called it the "higher forces" that serve.

Those forces are only available here and now. So, what's keeping you awake now? In its terror or excitement, be with it in recognition of its higher service. When you cultivate an internal environment that welcomes all that occurs to you, you will attract opportunities in trusting alliance with your thoughts. Seemingly tragic events will unfurl their purpose and become fertile ground for a new harvest.

SHIFTING PERSPECTIVE

Take out a journal and divide a blank page in half. Label one column with "Outer" and the other column with "Inner." Under the first column, write down, without too much pause, as many things, events, or people that make you feel like the world is coming at you. These are what consequently make you feel victimized or disconnected from your own sense of control. When you've exhausted the space in this column, pause and reflect on the items. Now, take the time to list each item's corresponding inner

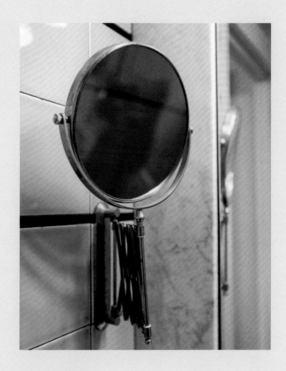

reflection under the second column. Here, write down aspects of control or shifts in perspective that you have regarding this situation or person. Sit in the reminder that even at times where we seemingly lack control over our lives, we have a choice in the way we approach and shape our worldview of it.

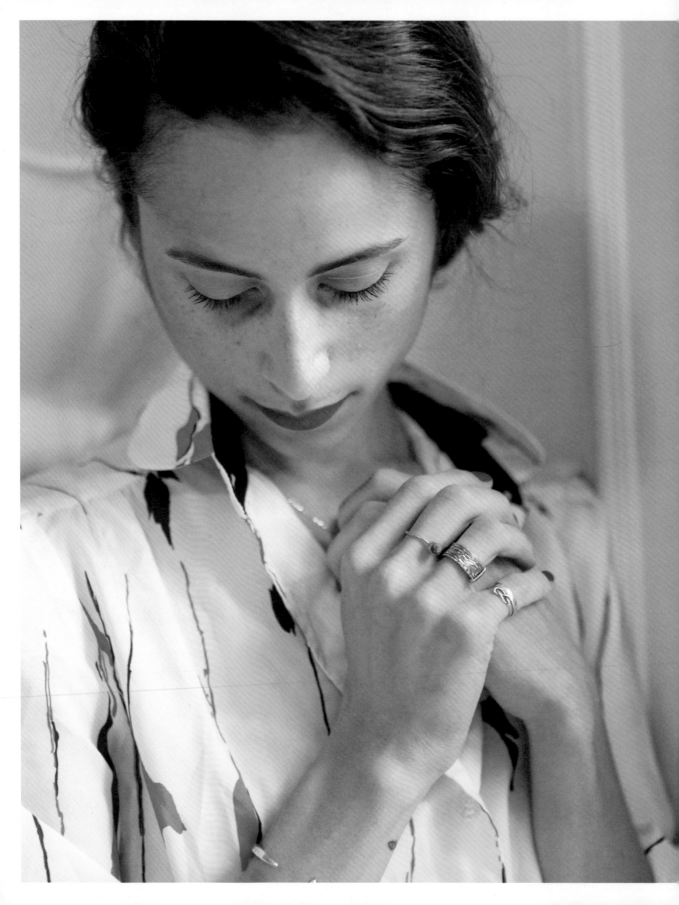

REDEFINING PRAYER

If you pray or meditate, how do you carry it along with you when you rise from the pew, your meditation cushion, or lower your hands? Is prayer a task or a single point in the day to prick your ears? How do you listen throughout the rest of your day?

If praying or meditating is not a practice for you, what keeps you from it? Stripped of any religious or spiritual association, what would prayer or meditation mean to you? To whom or what would you be connecting?

A prayer or meditation is not a set practice that we take in and out of a container held by the bounds of time, space, or doctrines. Instead, it's a way to pay careful attention to something besides ourselves, our judgements, and our preconceptions. Prayer is a declaration, a communication of our thoughts and desires for not just ourselves but for others. The Hebrew prophet Isaiah said, "My word shall not return unto me void, but shall accomplish that which it is sent to do." Our thoughts take on a form of energetic conversation where there is always a reaction to its action.

In its essence, then, prayer is a medium for paying concentrated attention to our surroundings and our relationships, and for being in constant relation to them. It's a way to heighten our awareness of what we call upon ourselves and wish upon others. May we redefine what prayer means to us with the intention of making every observance and interaction a prayer.

KNOW THIS

Prayer in Its Various Forms

All of these seemingly minute or regularly occurring events in our lives can have a profound and surprising depth to them when we give them prayerful attention:

- Taking a walk or hike in nature, especially after rain or snowfall
- Any physical activity, such as running, swimming, or yoga
- Mindfulness-based stress reduction (MBSR) or meditation
- Enjoying a cup of tea alone in the morning
- Spending time with loved ones or friends, away from technology
- Taking a shower or bath

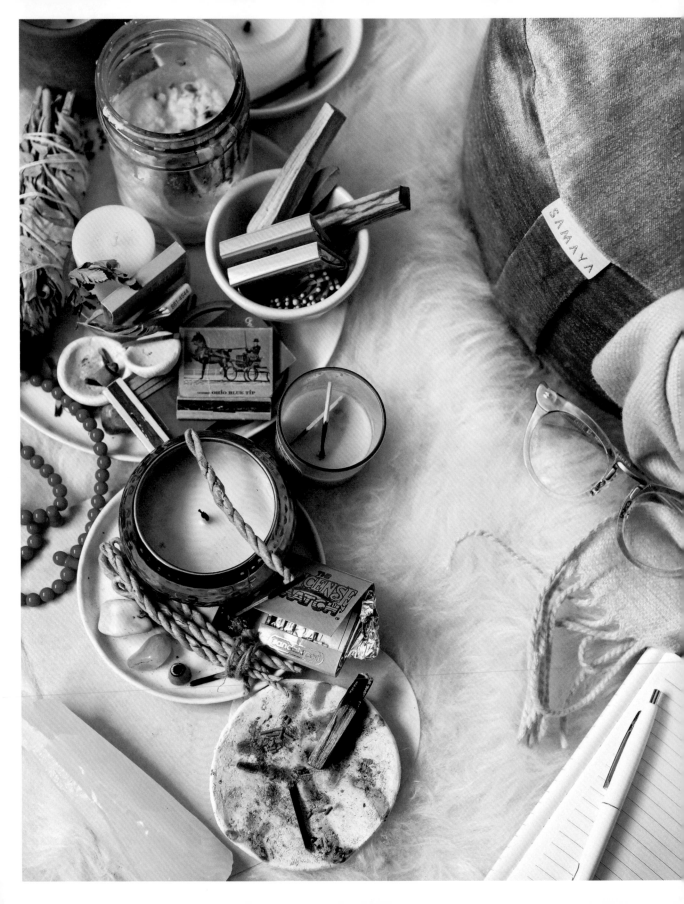

ele

OFF THE CUSHION MEDITATION

Sitting down for meditation is a practice in and of itself. Once you are seated, meditation is anything but a predictable, static activity. For creatures of habit like myself, this basic understanding of meditation is what makes a daily practice both challenging and comforting. There is the pleasure of depending on a structured time in the day for meditation, but also the trepidation of facing the thoughts that have arisen from the events of a new day. Meditation is dynamic and unknown, mirroring the primary fear most of us have in thinking of the future.

This also stems from our tendency to view our day-to-day tasks as a list of chores: dry brush, check; breakfast, check; run, check; head to pillow, check. Panic strikes when we close our eyes and sleep doesn't arrive on time. We're either rushing toward something or picking at our hangnails in an impatient spiral of thoughts waiting for something or someone. But meditation isn't just another chore on your schedule. It's a reserved time that makes the rest of our time more efficient. Not every day is going to necessitate an 11-minute meditation, while some days will demand longer sits. Sometimes just finding the time to sit can lead to a meditation on feeling overwhelmed—are you overcommitted in your schedule or to others? Where are *you* within your priorities?

Make yourself worth a minute and make mundane tasks a meditation. Take your meditation off the cushion and the clock. When you heat a kettle for tea, listen to the water boil. When you brush your teeth, feel your gums, your teeth, the flavor of the paste, and the quality of your grip on the toothbrush. Meditate on sensations.

When you find yourself the time to sit down, don't time your meditation. Allow your mind to guide you through what it needs and for how long. Observe what arises when your heart guides your meditation rather than your watch.

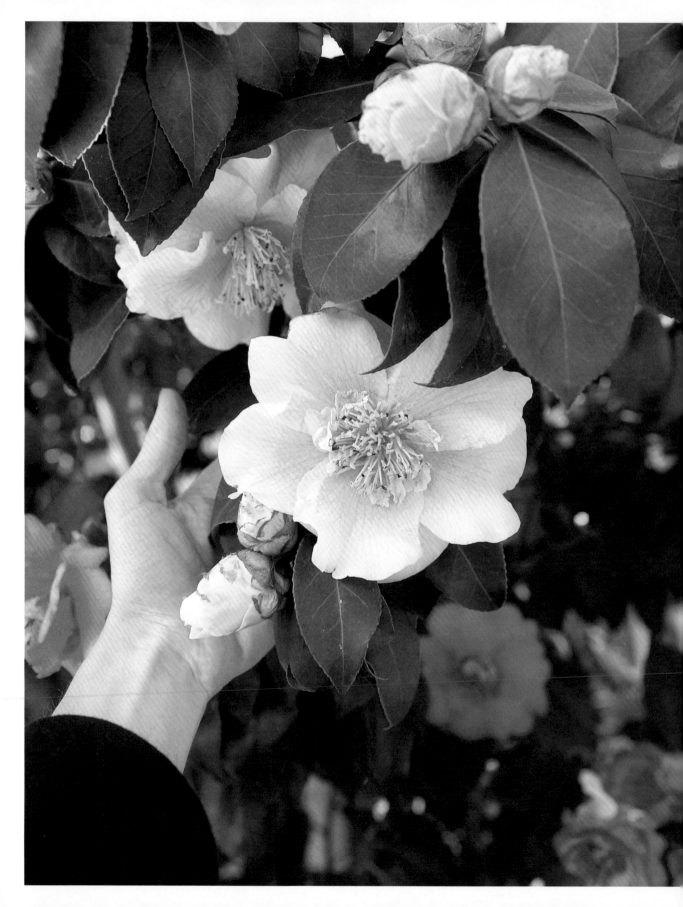

ele

COURAGE IN LE CŒUR

"Courage" is the arrangement of the heart, *le cœur*, over the mind in relation to what is faced. When you are positioned against your fears, how do you arrange yourself? Do you approach the unknown only through the validation or compass of another? Or do you face it from your personal viewpoint, becoming a green light to guide you through your own waters?

Speak to yourself as you would with a friend, whether over afternoon tea or a sullen shoulder. Both extremes of life—the casual delights and its merciless heart-in-throat pangs—require courage. And this courage rises with the settling of the heart that comes in time. To have courage: cœur / age . . . heavy in the heart, not as a drag but in its knowledge of where it stands, with the confidence that where you are and where you are going are driven by *you*, rather than dragged at the heels of another. Courage is to walk toward the unknown by kneeling at its feet.

You are your own solider, your own commander—lead your own way.

CHATTR CHAKKR VARTEE

Chant the following kundalini mantra to dispel fear of the unknown, instill courage, and command.

Chattr chakkr vartee
Chattr chakkr bhugatay
Suyumphay suphang sarab daa sarab jugtay
Dukaalang pranaasee dayaalang saroopay
Sadaa ung sungay aphangang biphootay

Thou art pervading in all the four directions, the Enjoyer in all the four directions.
Thou art self-illuminated and united with all.
Destroyer of bad times, embodiment of mercy.
Thou art ever within us.
Thou are the everlasting giver of un-destroyable power.

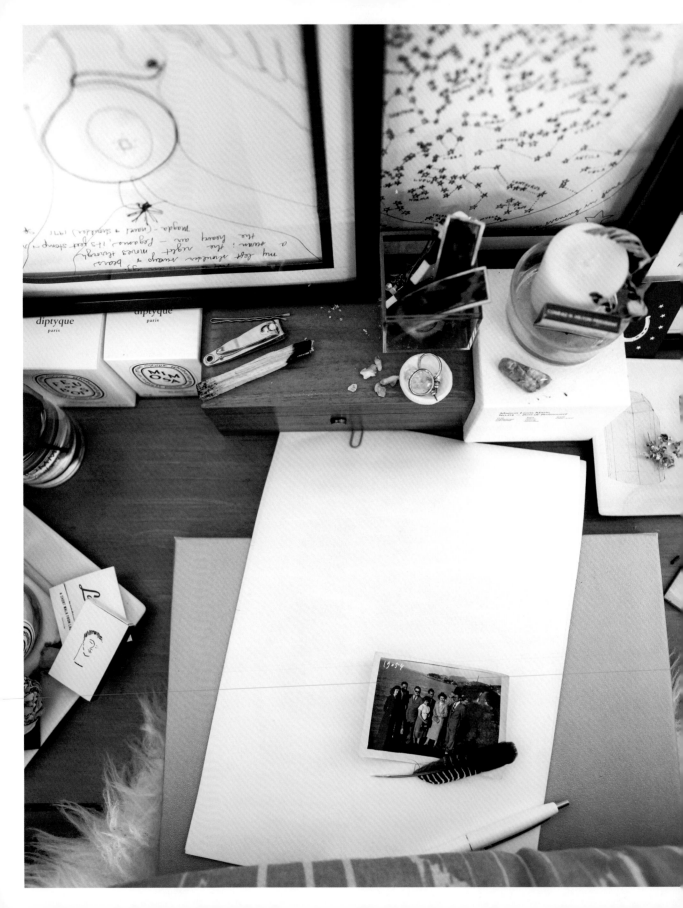

LOVING LIST

Often when we catch ourselves thinking or speaking negatively, we clench in guilt but then ignore it. Our body, however, registers this reaction on a cellular and subconscious level. These low-level perspectives and reactions become a catalyst for future low-level perspectives and reactions that attract negative energy to ourselves.

Feeling guilty about money or feeling like you don't have enough, for example, cannot attract abundance. Even when there are limited resources, we must spend with gratitude that the money we have is serving us. We must give when we can and revel in the joy of karmic abundance. If your finances are *the* topic that dampens your spirits and causes you to spew out negative words, as is the case for many, work to shift your thought process on money first (page 113).

Even minor negative thoughts such as frustration over a partner or roommate's unwashed dishes have deep roots. In sour interactions, observe the levels of communication. Have you been expressing your emotions clearly and has the other as well? How are you listening to each other? Even when we listen, we do so through our own filters and the stories we've spun about and around others. If you notice that the person with whom you're interacting is expressing an issue, emotion, or dilemma, repeat what you hear back to them to clear up and avoid misunderstandings. When we can achieve that level ground in our relationships, we can make space for ourselves to hold attention for others.

To do so, take the time to create a list that you gradually curate over a few days. Jot down habitual negative thoughts, reactions, and interactions. Then list the opposite, loving form you would like to transform each negative feeling into.

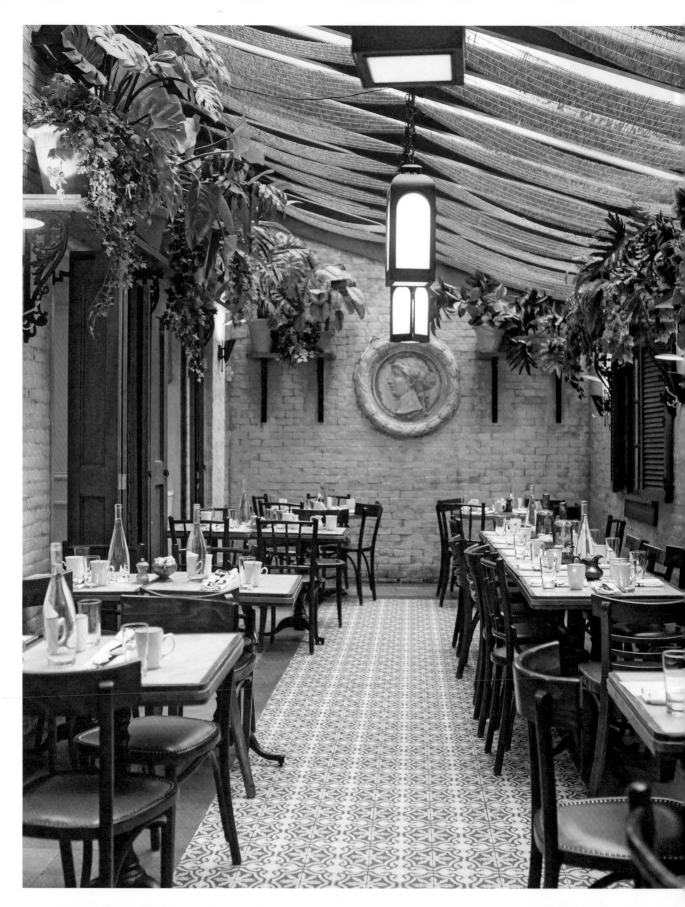

MENTAL FURNITURE

In the glimmer of the Information Age, our minds are slowly coming to resemble the cotton- and soap-smelling muted living room of a grandmother—reeking of slow energy and movement. Swiping down to refresh social media platforms, our eyes dart at our forgotten book or stare into the memory of meditation. At work, we force ourselves to not pick up (or rather click on) a calculator to plug in elementary arithmetic problems. We're all hopping or tripping amidst one mental dust bunny or another, weaving cobwebs in our minds, overly dependent on technology. So, here's to rising from the dust. This is a commitment to re-engage muscular memory and re-invigorate the mind.

Exercising the mind is as important as exercising the body. Delightfully, there are as many mental workouts as there are physical ones. Open yourself to regularly playing memorization or problem-solving games. This can be anything from sudoku and crossword puzzles to memorizing a poem. A professor at Columbia University called this kind of memorization investing in your own "mental furniture." He had memorized many of Shakespeare's sonnets, and found comfort in how their words settled themselves in his mind like furniture for his thoughts to sit on through his life. Dust off your mental pillows now so your thoughts can rest in rich repose in your later years.

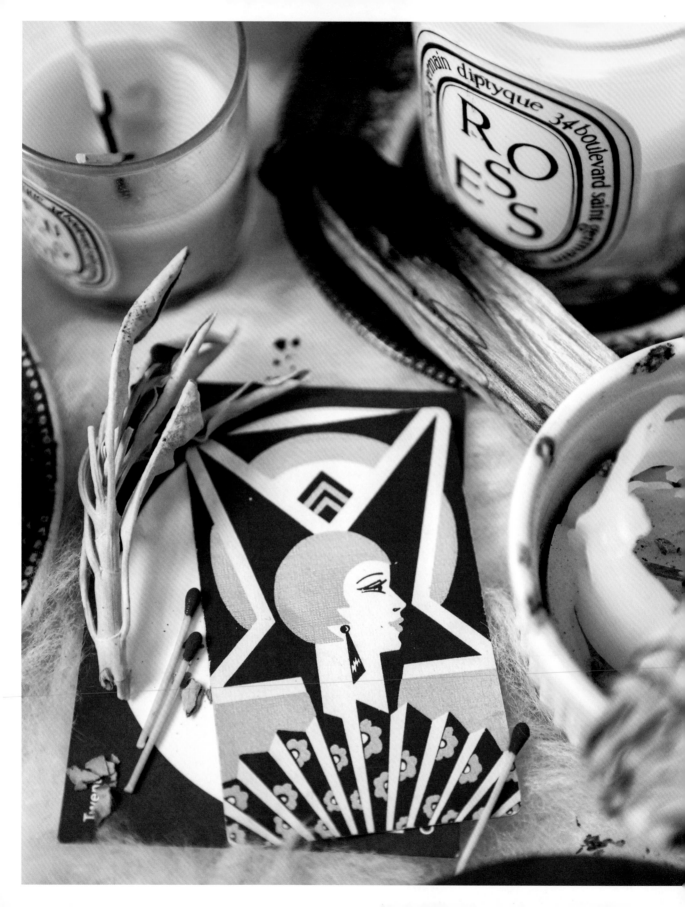

GADGETS & GIZMOS

The White Rabbit from *Alice's Adventures in Wonderland* is a spirit animal to many—we're always in a rush. There is neither a party for which we might be due nor are we in a stew, and we're rarely ever late! Yet, we're always in a hurry. There is a running joke about my fast-paced walking, that I look like I'm on a mission even if I'm just getting a glass of water. I'll sip it and arrive at a meeting, probably twenty minutes early. *Why the hurried footsteps and a rushed heart?*

I have observed this not only with my physical engagements; I'm also running around in my mind. Most of us feel this way, enmeshed within this digital microcosm. There is an onslaught of information: 0.62 seconds to load 471,000,000 articles; Netflix is not loading, let's hop on over to Instagram; oh, a notification from Facebook; emails equivalent to a stack of papers; too many browser tabs open to read their names . . .

What are you doing? Are you here in the now or are you plotting in a half-sketched version of your future self? Slow down your steps in order to step into the present moment, which is all that is happening. In the present, you are evolving. In your own presence, you download the energy of the Universe into yourself rather than the distractions of your gadgets and gizmos. The urge to reach for our phones is a desire to feed an unfulfilled ego, especially in comparison to the online presence of others—what are they doing and getting that we don't have? It's a rabbit hole of a habit, leaving us feeling more disconnected than ever.

Exiting this spiral pushes us to have our own code bank to rely on, to construct a new language out of our own here and now. It's not a prescription to completely detach ourselves from the lure of technology, but rather a small stepping away. Jot down how many times you resort to checking social media. With eyes likely wide open at the number you end up with, consider why you turn to social media so frequently—is it a form of procrastination? Are you fending off anxiety about how to approach a task? If these questions make you miss your social media, try instead to meditate for five minutes to center your attention and focus, or ask a friend for help with the task. This will then not only lessen your technological habits and associated anxieties, but you will also feel good about getting things done.

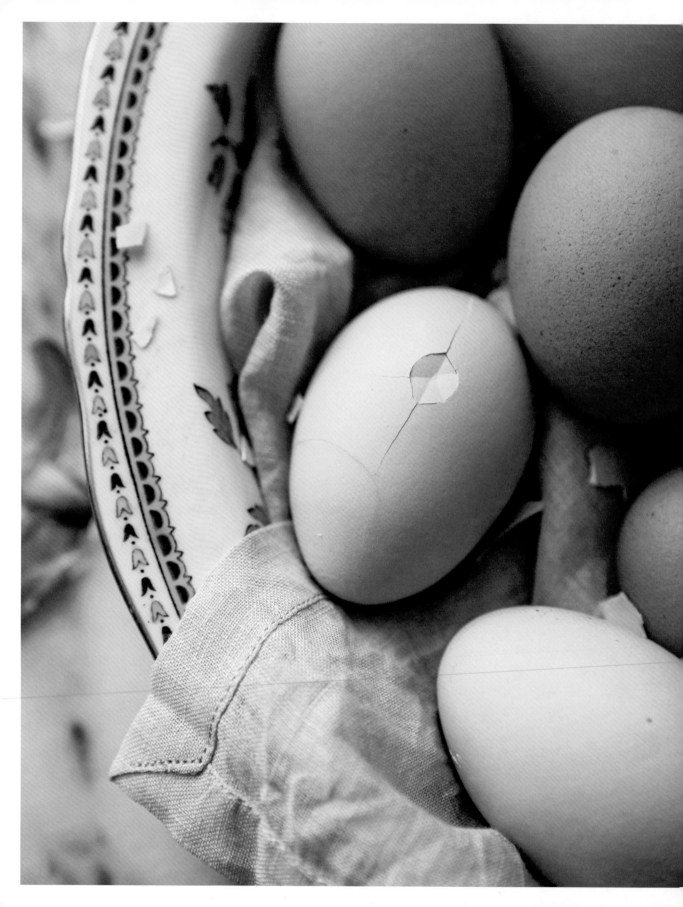

THE CRACK

Our emotions are a dainty platter heaped with eggs. Each egg is like a container of shielded thoughts, unspoken words, and tender emotions, encased in a fragile shell against the view of another.

When one of your eggs cracks, what comes oozing out? Is what you contain within yourself a mirror of your presentation to the world? Or are you cocooned inside a sticky suspension, the crack on the shell revealing a slit of hidden thoughts, expressions, and judgements you can't swim through.

Are you surprised at what has been harboring within the neat shell? Or have you been sitting on the warming familiarity of your veiled emotions, secretly bearing a darker you on a nest of entangled thoughts?

As an egg inevitably cracks, so do our emotions, whether they're buried or arranged perfectly for display. And out of a crack comes a birth of another you. The yolk may have split in the break—it's no perfect presentation. When we hide our emotions from others, we also conceal them from ourselves. How we are viewed by others is a direct reflection of how we face ourselves. A crack in your shell is an opportunity for you to notice what you've been hiding so that you can become whole again. Then turn to dust your broken shell and bury it in new fertile ground to walk upon. A rebirth.

THE SHIELD MEDITATION

You might find from time to time that, despite attentive self-care or because of a lack thereof, your energy is drained. It might resemble the feeling of being contained within a cracked eggshell with the sap of your energy oozing out. In such cases or as part of a regular energetic shielding routine, practice this simple meditation. Position yourself comfortably either on a meditation cushion, a chair, or lying down. Allow yourself for the first two minutes to pace your breath according to its natural rhythm—don't try to change or deepen it.

Slowly shift your focus to your heart-center as you imagine a ball of light in the middle of your chest. Imagine it gradually increasing in size, following the rhythm of your breath. Patiently see this ball of light growing in size to eventually create an entire shield of light around you. Visualize the rays around it, the warm center right in your chest, and its dynamic flow as you breathe. Sit or lie down for as long as you'd like, basking in the comfort that this light will be shielding you through and out of your meditation in your daily life.

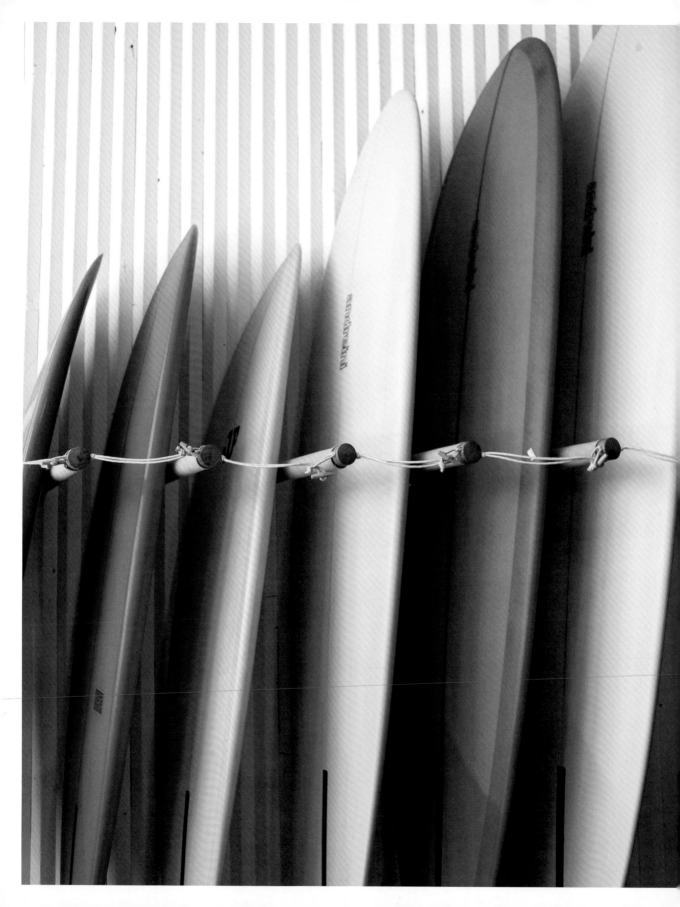

MOMENTOUS MOMENTUM

Are you driving or being driven? Is your drive merely the momentum of the car or your own foot on the pedal? When we head towards a certain goal, we may find ourselves unconsciously coasting toward it rather than steadily trucking with a plan towards our goal. Without a set pace and plan, we might find ourselves speeding to our desired destination, swerving from one lane to another of directions we could possibly take. We could find ourselves in a tunnel of unforeseen visions and hallucinations of what ought to be, distracted from our real vision. Our goal consequently can become a mere hazy glow at the end—a rosy vision to look at but which is out of our reach. In pursuit of your destination, what is it that you are leaving behind and heading towards?

As we go about our daily lives, we can sometimes end up on a detour, especially if we're the ones being driven, rather than doing the driving. This could land us on a dirt road pebbled with the skeleton of an earlier version or forgotten part of ourselves. In our lives, as we move from one place to another—in our minds or around the globe—we're constantly being sent reminders of this past version of ourselves. If we're steady, if we're in the driver's seat, this won't send us off course. In fact, it can be useful to see where we've come from, how our aims have refined, shifted, and grown with us. Where we're less steady, we can get pulled into old currents.

A physical move from one location to another requires packing, and so does an an emotional one. Take the bow off the package of your vision and see its contents. To achieve a goal or growth, we must first unpack or face what we have been carrying over from the past. You may see your vision clearly, but what direction are your current actions actually propelling you towards? It takes practice, like working a muscle, to consistently align our day-to-day actions with our long- and short-term goals. Are you aligned or are your habits bound to break you away from what you've intended? What is motioning you towards your goal or of treading newfound lands?

To set out in a new direction, we must first engage the force that is driving us. We might be envisioning a new path not from the vantage point of steady ground or an understanding of where we are, but in the haste of where we want to be. Remember that urgency is just a feeling. It is only through careful reflection of the force behind our actions and desires—our true intentions—that we can achieve momentous momentum—a drive for and towards ourselves and what will ultimately serve us well.

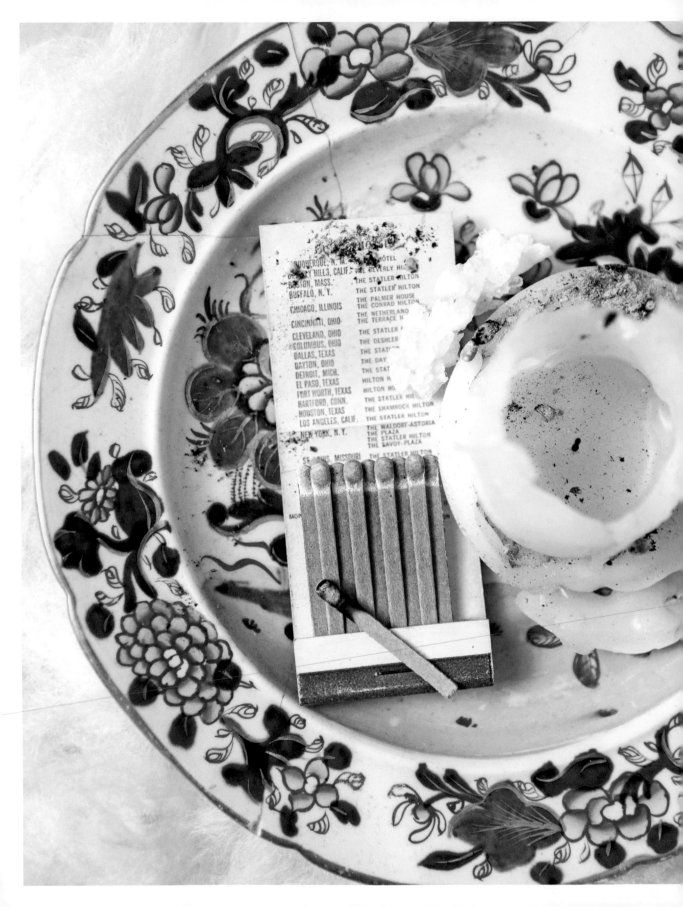

SELFLESS SELFISHNESS

Are you here and now with yourself or are you flinging yourself into the future through a trajectory of always saying "yes" to others? On the dawn of that tomorrow, who are you rising for and how many times have you said "no" to yourself to say "yes" to someone else, leaving yourself in the dust? Are you being honest in your time and commitment to yourself?

In the teetering balance between external needs and obligations and internal ones, shift a greater balance toward your internal interactions; focus on selfcare. Create fluidity between yourself and your surroundings. When we allow ourselves the flow of our own time, we also permit others to drift through theirs.

Amidst a schedule that flings your time here and there, reel it back to yourself without confused feelings of selfishness. When someone asks for your time, take the time to think about it, to say "I don't know," or dare to say "no." You can say "no" to others—to your loved ones even—without withdrawing from love. Rather, saying "no" signifies love in its honesty toward others about your condition and ability to provide. And an automatic, unthinking "yes" isn't always a sign of love. Fulfilling expectations should fill you with energy, not drain you. "Yes" should not be an obligation but a sign of care, for both you and the other. May you redefine saying "no" as learning to say "yes" to yourself.

VERBAL
SELF-AWARENESS

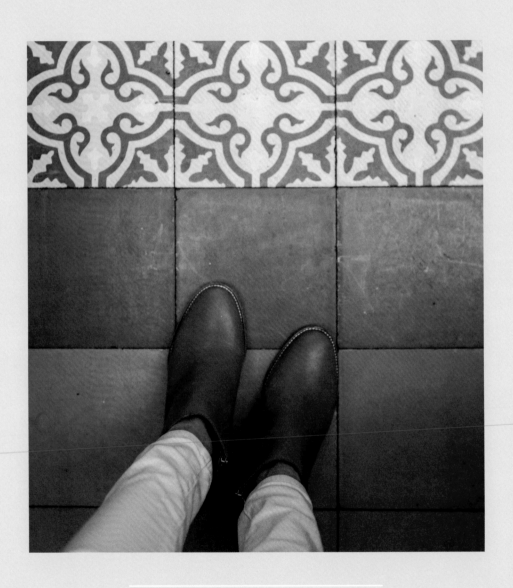

Our words have a powerful effect on both ourselves and others. In cultivating attentive conversations with others, we must begin with ourselves. When we do not speak within and for ourselves, we not only create a pattern of destruction in ourselves but also in others as they struggle to create a narrative of assumed causes for our behaviors. A nonexistent or inarticulate inner dialogue leads to either miscommunication or misinformation.

This generally leads to retraction or its complete opposite: a tearful conversation on tangential issues in avoidance of the actual matter at hand. Rather than unraveling a complexity of emotions, these verbal tangents create an unresolved imprint of yet another traumatic misunderstanding of our emotions. Emotions become repeatedly seen as undervalued, incomprehensible, and blocking connection with others. We consequently spin ourselves into a web of thoughts out of the stories we assume people are weaving about us.

We then wander, tilt, and shift between polar ends of the emotional spectrum. Caught in small talk, we either mutter out our unhappy states in a deep haze of work or exclaim mechanically "I'm good" and "How do you do?" through smiles that disappear behind backs. We either retract into our work or pretend we are happily floating above it all.

Instead, allow yourself to listen to your feelings when they emerge rather than wilting in their burning honesty. Acknowledge and speak to them. This is a process of processing. We must see ourselves, must communicate and face our egos, and untangle the untruths we tell ourselves about ourselves in order to communicate with our external world. Inquire within. Cultivate awareness of how your utterances and actions differ from your inner narratives. Tell on yourself, point your finger at your fears, and untangle the mesh that you have veiled yourself behind.

Acknowledge your emotions rather than allowing yourself to be paralyzed in fear of past experiences or trapped in habitual reactions. Greet your anger, your sadness, your defenses. Attempt to locate their origin not only to comprehend your reactions but also to value your negative emotions and forgive yourself for having them.

Everyone has their own narrative that causes deeply imprinted habitual emotional reactions. Tracing the trajectory of your emotional roots, you will be able to lift the emotional walls that no longer serve their purpose so that you can return to your best self. Take the sweet time to hear and honor your own stories so you may lend an empathetic ear to those of others.

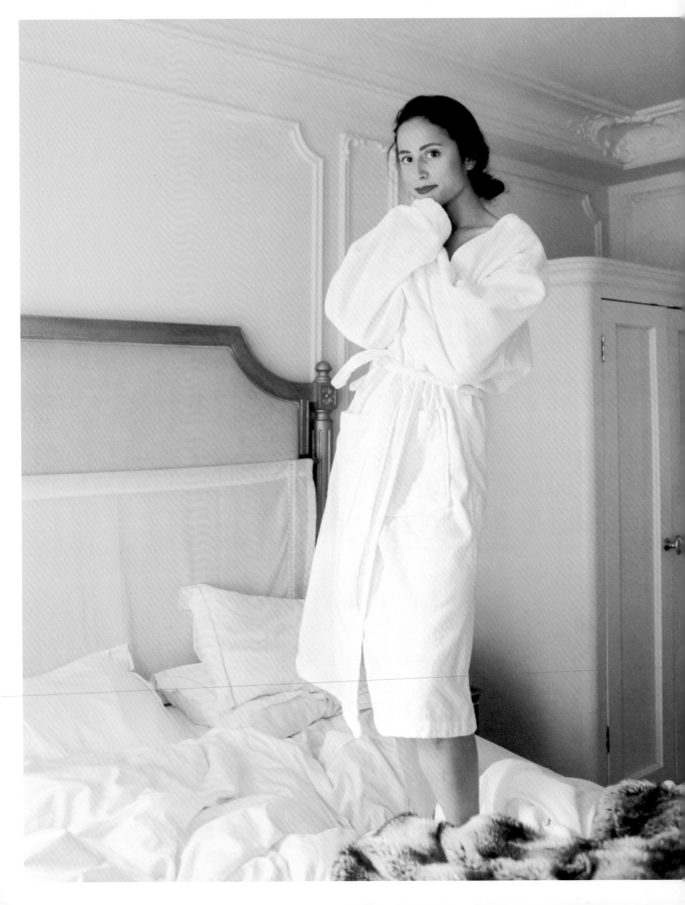

BODY TALK

For many of us, we rarely connect the physical body with our spiritual and emotional bodies. This lack of alignment leads to energy imbalances that can manifest in a variety of ways, such as emotionally with angry outbursts or physically with tension headaches.

To realign the bodies, we must increase body awareness. This consciousness is not simply a matter of thought but also action. It's not a one-time, static performance but a continuous exercise of simultaneously learning from and teaching our bodies to forge a relationship between our emotions and actions. When we reconnect with our body, we increase awareness of our patterns, attitudes, and thoughts to empower ourselves.

When was the last time you intentionally looked at yourself naked? Not before a shower or undressing, but truly observed your body?

Set aside an hour in a room with a full-length mirror where you can be alone. Remove all clothing and jewelry. Stand in front of the mirror and observe what being nude generates for you. Do you feel uncomfortable and, if so, with what? Do you feel compelled to cover certain parts of your body and how so? Are there particular areas that feel tense? Do you see yourself as attractive? If not, by what yardstick or ideal are you measuring yourself? Who established this ideal? Other women, you, men, the media, childhood trauma? Do you allow yourself the right to look at yourself naked?

Deepen the conversation and start to discover your body head to toe by touching yourself, starting at the scalp. How does your own touch feel? Talk out loud to each part, such as "My freckles have increased. I enjoy them because they make me feel closer to my mother." The more deeply you create a conversation with your body, the more attuned you will become to where it holds emotional tension that can be released physically with a massage (page 60). Our entire body is a brain, storing memories, emotions, and beliefs in its tissues. Long after an accident, the body will continue to react to its trauma and release protective signals that cause the area tension. Body awareness reformats the language in which the body approaches its parts and faults, increasing circulation and vitality through renewed perspective.

UNCONTAINED EMOTIONS

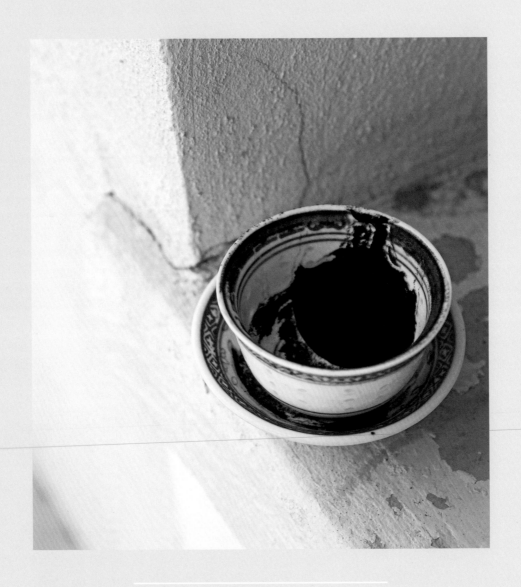

Integrative healer Dr. Habib Sadeghi refers to our internal state as a spiritual ecosystem. He further states that when women, the birthers and nurturers of humanity, are unable to nurture themselves, that emotional landscape dries up. We are increasingly exposed to life's tensions and traumas, further depleting our self-nourishing capabilities. Eventually, our internal state resembles that of a *Grapes of Wrath* scene—a dustbowl devoid of emotional food to nourish either the resident—ourselves—or others. Consequently, we store the emotional responses to our negative life experiences without the tools to tend to them. We live on the edge of our emotions ready to burst.

Renowned psychoanalyst Wilfred Bion called this particular state of emotional existence *uncontained*. According to his theory, thoughts or emotions are imbued with either a receptive, female quality or a projective, male one of underlying, subconscious responses. Powerful, articulated emotions in this case are not ones spoken by the quiet tongues of women and unheard minorities. Those equipped with the appropriate emotional outlets live in a state of uncontained emotions that allows for the release of emotions such as anger or resentment. While the receptive person, often a female, is stuck in a stasis of withholding emotions or thoughts.

When we release an uncontained emotion, it's a cry to have another see, hear, and hold space for us. Here, we can see the archetype of mother or woman again. This emotional cycle is rooted in childhood, where the mother functions as a "container" for the infant. She holds raw psychic material—thoughts, emotions, spiritual pain—acknowledges it, and endows it with meaning. She essentially metabolizes or breaks apart the raw effects so the child can then *digest* their emotions appropriately. Eventually, the child learns through this cycle to reflect on her own sensations and emotional experiences independently.

Unfortunately, not many adults become their own container. Hauled by uncontained emotions that surround them, they either politely bottle them up or release them through external stimulations, addictions, self-harm, or even crime. Women deplete themselves to the point of uncontained emotions by prioritizing caring for others over themselves.

As Dr. Sadeghi observes, this takes a toll on women's bodies; out of the 23.5 million Americans who suffer from autoimmune disease, 75 percent of them are women according to the National Institute of Health (NIH) with a 10:1 ratio of Hashimoto's thyroiditis, 7:1 of Grave's disease, and 9:1 of lupus.

A festering of buried emotions bruises our system, creating dis-ease in the body. We strive to meditate in the morning, eat breakfast, get promoted at work, get drinks with friends, but also detox, do yoga, *and* run the extra physical mile so we can avoid that nightcap of judging ourselves for inadequacy, or not running the extra metaphorical mile.

We need to remember that emotions are emotions, neither good nor evil. They all equally need to be acknowledged, voiced or processed, and released. This is a guide to feel your feelings and be a container for yourself. It's about the feminine, of letting go and trusting our intuition. And when you cannot, call on another. Help is humbling.

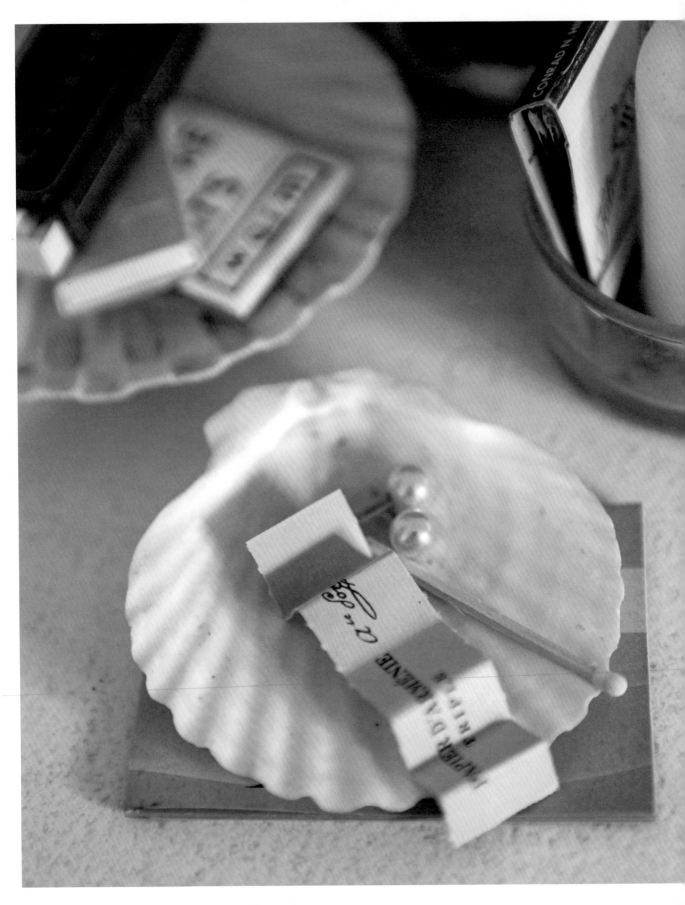

SORRY BUT THANK YOU

In the breaking of a date or an unfashionably late arrival, how do you greet others? When you compose a belated email, how do you begin? Eyebrows furrowed and fingers twisted in guilt, do you apologize in profuse synonyms of "I'm sorry?" What tone do you set for others to react to the situation? Do you allow them to see and empathize with your chaotic state? Or are you starting things off on a sour note where you either increase the irritation of the other or create it with your self-incrimination?

Excessively apologizing is a habitual tendency for many, born out of a Puritan ethic that makes us feel guilt over situations out of our control. We feel sorry for ourselves, sorry for the state we're in, sorry for putting another in that state, and sorry for being so sorry.

Others around us feel this cycle of low-level vibration. Rather than feeling pleasure from an apology, they instead feel the discomfort of this stagnated energy. As a result, meetings begun this way have static communication, and feel restricted and stiff.

It takes only a minor shift to establish a softer pattern. We can acknowledge the inconvenience that we might have caused others in a positive way rather than muttering low-tone apologies. Instead of immediately apologizing, thank the other person for their patience. Let them know that you are aware of and cherish the time they have given to you. Thank them for their generosity in a world where time is not liberal and some days are not kind yet we can be so towards one another.

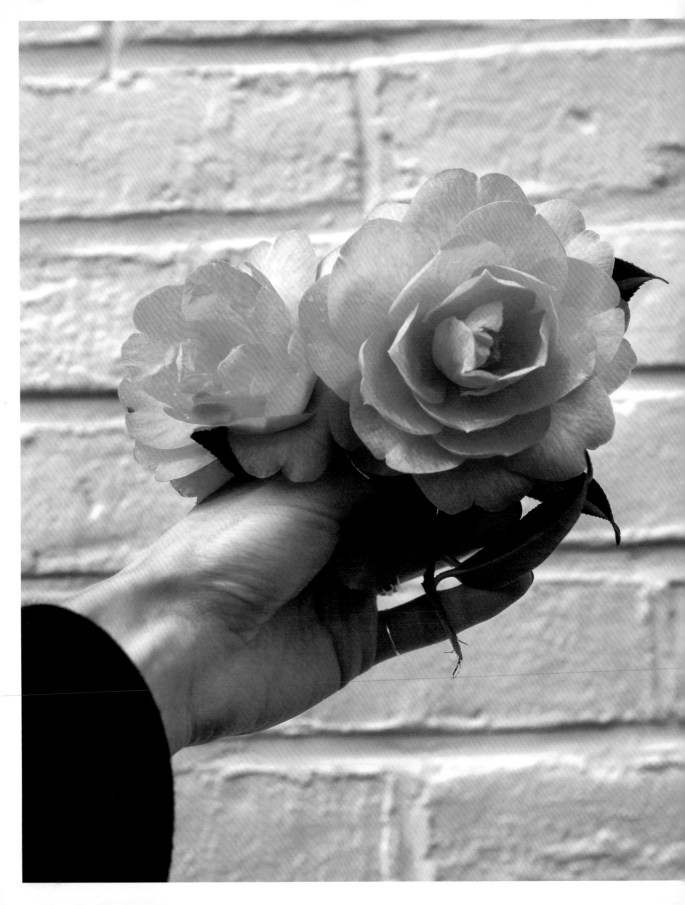

DO-OVERS

Generally, when we apologize, we see the apology as the conclusion of an argument or conversation—an apology as period. Yet how many times have you said, "I'm sorry," just to hush over your feelings and thoughts? Does your story become a whisper in the utterance of your apology? How can you listen to the other without silencing yourself?

An apology is for the other *and* for you. For the other, it is a recognition of the treatment they desire and deserve. A lifting of your hands away from your ears, of hearing again. For yourself, it is a simultaneous witnessing of your mistake and your acknowledgement of it—a see something, say something. And now you're listening, two ears perked for two—hearing not only your own story but that of the other. This is where a do-over comes in, a practice to tune into unsaid words and emotions.

Home and family dynamics is a fitting scenario. Often, when we come home from work, we are on edge from the day's stresses or obligations. These make our emotions into matches that the smallest thing or act by our partner, roommate, or family member can strike. To be greeted by dirty laundry on the floor, for instance, can spark an equally immediate response of angry criticism.

While there may not be a logical reason to explain the mess, there is almost never one for an angry, presumptuous response. We realize this as we, or after we, blurt out our criticism. Take this moment to offer a do-over. State the reason why it caused you anger, that you should not have reacted as such, and ask for the acceptance of your apology. Ask for a do-over and listen to the other's explanation of the issue.

⚯

CONSCIOUSNESS RAISING GROUPS

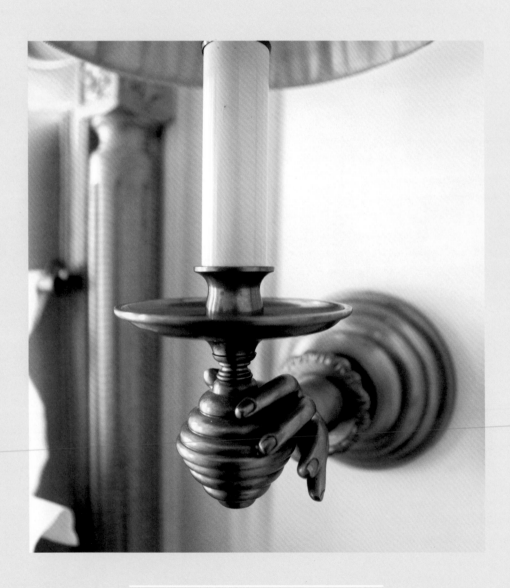

"... Our feelings are telling us something from which we can learn. . . that our feelings mean something worth analyzing . . . that our feelings are saying something *political*."

—KATHIE SARACHILD

Consciousness-raising (C-R) is a tool that originated in the 1960s by the Women's Liberation Movement to "tell it like it is." It was a gathering against the isolation mid-century feminists were feeling as women. They argued that many issues in women's lives were consequently misidentified as experiential ones between single women and men rather than systemic forms of oppression. Raising consciousness thus meant sharing feelings and experiences to expand self awareness and consequently political awareness.

Then and now, C-R groups can cultivate a better grasp of women's oppression by speaking of its experiences and holding it by its tongue. Leading from feelings into political action, we can understand and shatter the plight of the women's condition.

This model calls for a shift in attitude, from the passive hushing or complaining to assertive speaking, acting, and challenging. It's a gathering to share without interference or fear, without man-woman hierarchy or even amongst women. It's a way to realize that one woman's achievement does not mean another woman's failure, that we can share in our success and knowledge gained.

To start a C-R group, gather a small number of women, some of whom you know, others you don't. Do this with a friend or two, with each person picking a few acquaintances. Limit the size to no more than twelve to gather informally at a member's home or another safe space.

At the first meeting, gather in a circle and allow people to introduce themselves and their reason for being there. Define the place, frequency at which the group will meet, and the duration of each meeting. Allow the group to be "leaderless" with the whole group taking responsibility for its existence, which prevents anyone from "mothering" the group.

Be mindful that the aim of a C-R group is to share and not to advise or solve problems, which can also create a "mothering" effect and are often rooted in structural oppression. Instead, *listen*. Relate to one another's personal problems, identify larger cultural issues, and perhaps conjure up community actions. Most importantly, validate one another's experiences as women.

Do not resist speaking or bitching about the oppressors in your life. If feelings of guilt consequently arise, discuss why the need to be hushed and thus protect them arises. Pick a different topic each week, such as the ones from the questions below inspired by the Chicago Women's Libration Union (CWLU) Herstory Project, and share your reactions.

How do you think men or other women view you?
Do you have a preference over having a girl or
    boy child?
How do you feel about housework and your
    partner's duties?
What has kept you from doing what you'd like
    to in life?
What is being feminine?
How do you feel about menstruation and when you
    had your first one?
What did you learn about sex from your parents?
How do you define a "good girl"?
Do you feel pressured to like or bear children and
    by whom?

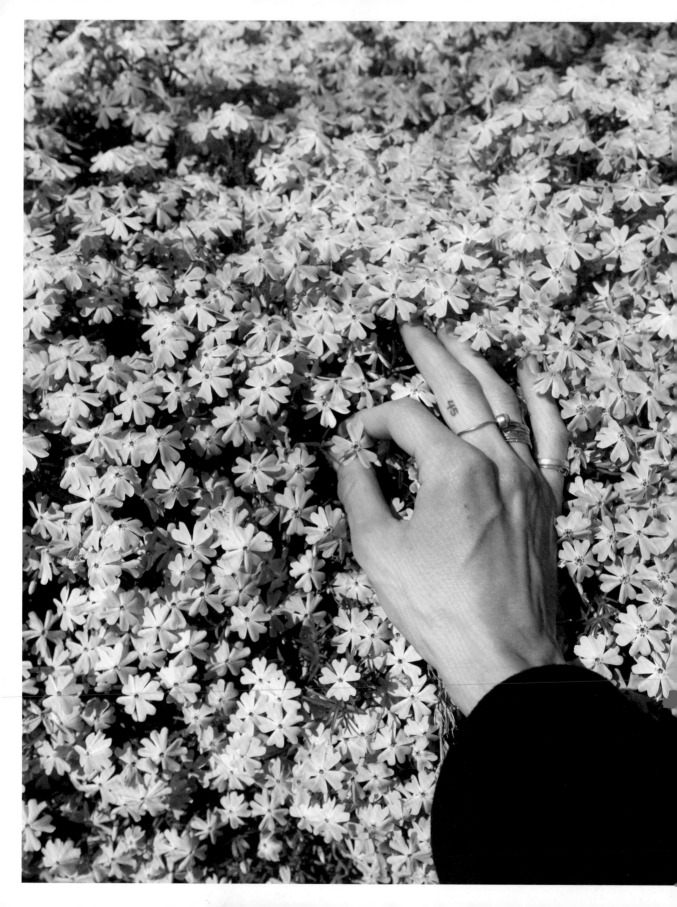

PULLING OUR WEIGHT

A labored minute, an hour carved out of patterned habits, touchstones of fear, and a narrow vision. Whatever dirt road of life we're traveling on, we will only continue to cloud our vision into a dust bowl when we allow our feet to be dragged by fear.

In settling the dust and into ourselves, let's pull our own weight, owning our part in the pattern rather than being dragged by it. Let's observe how we pave our own road and our level of participation in carving out the journey of others. Relinquish the control of our own outcomes and those of others so we can responsibly carry the weight of only our own.

We are free to choose the way in which we ascribe meaning to circumstances in our lives. The same applies to allowing such freedom for others. As David Foster Wallace said, letting go of managing another's condition is to "truly care about other people and to sacrifice for them, over and over, in myriad petty little unsexy ways, every day."[2]

When we attempt to pave the path of others, to steer them in the direction dictated by our own vision, we weigh both parties down. Let's let ourselves and others swim in the waters of that freedom.

BREATHWORK FOR SELF-CONTROL

At times when we feel the obligations and responsibilities we have for our loved ones weighing a little too heavily, we can depend on this meditation. Its sheer simplicity and repetition renders a monotone quality to the dynamic, racing thoughts we often experience. It allows the mind to focus instead on the rhythmic repetitions, allowing us to feel a sense of control through our own breath to remind us to pull our weight for ourselves.

Position yourself comfortably either on a meditation cushion, a chair, or lying down. Allow yourself for the first two minutes to pace your breathing according to its natural rhythm—don't try to change or deepen it. When you feel that your breath is steady and calm, slowly begin to inhale from your belly to the count of four. When you reach the top of your breath, exhale to the count of eight. Repeat this set ten times, or for longer if necessary to achieve a sense of balance.

WOMAN TO WOMAN

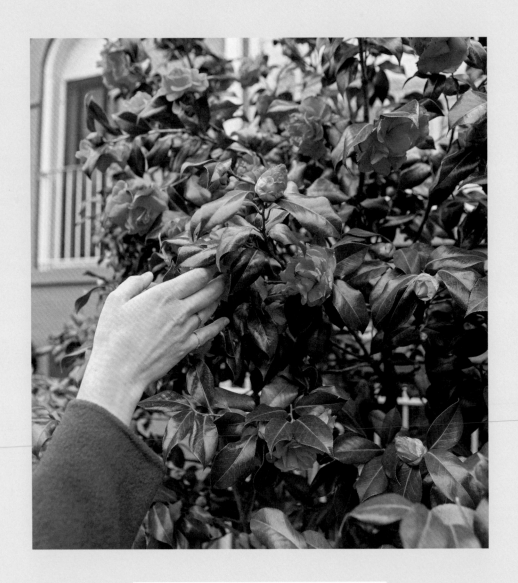

How do you relate to other women? How do you relate to yourself as a woman? Our treatment of ourselves teaches others how to treat us. The emotions or perspectives that we cultivate toward ourselves reflect not only our state of self-identity but also how we view other women.

How do you feel when your partner interacts with other women? Do you feel threatened? If you do feel discomfort, why does it arise from the other woman rather than your partner? Often we feel that certain women possess something that we don't. How does this external comparison reflect upon how you internally value yourself? Observe if it creates a sense of lack that has been engrained or merely prompted by comparison.

Similarly, notice where you locate your sexuality. Do you consider women to be less sexual or erotic than men? Consider how you define masculinity and femininity. Do you judge other women in regards to how "feminine" they are? Does this stem from an obligation you or other women feel in performing a certain "female" role? What social constructions or norms perpetuate this state and consequently separate you from connecting with other women?

We often find ourselves competing with other women primarily through these oppressive structures that perpetuate the imagery of being a "woman" or "female" as being dainty, sweet, polite, submissive, emotional, irrational, or even manic. On the other hand, men are often described as strong, independent, in control, in charge, and are even made to be attractive when they are considered "bad boys." How does your behavior align with these stereotypes? Do you consider being female interchangeable with being feminine? What adjectives do you use to describe yourself and are you attached to the approval you receive from these supposed feminine characteristics?

You will likely find that most feminine characteristics are neither a true reflection of yourself or the women you admire. Instead, they are boundaries that prevent women from displaying their intelligence, assertiveness, and voice, but also from being angry, sloppy, or unfair. Restricted by these societal norms and roles, many women either surrender their power to men or use it in devious, calculating ways that rob them of their values and connections to other women. In taking back our own power as women, we should not only experience it openly ourselves but also allow other women to do so. We can redefine what being female is in our relations with other women rather than as the "opposite" sex. We can remove ourselves from both the oppression of patriarchal norms and that of competition with other women. She is not to blame and doing so only diverts our energies from the source of injustice. To bask in the light of another woman does not make our own light dimmer. To see her as a model rather than a competitor allows us to reach for the rings of the ladder together, going up without letting each other down.

Try making a commitment to yourself, or having a personal policy, not to engage in gossip about other females. Practice regular self-appreciation, not as a woman but of your being and body; practice abhyanga (page 60) and mirror observations (page 99). Start with strengthening your bond to yourself as a woman and a human being to reflect that compassion unto others.

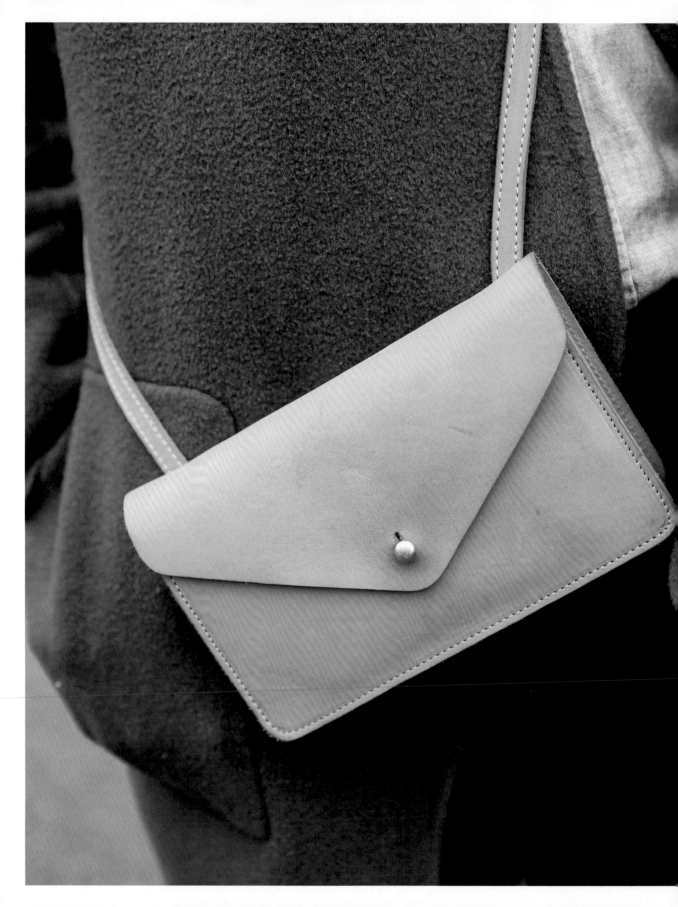

MONEY MATTERS

When you receive a paycheck or any sum of money, do you grip onto it in fear? When you purchase something for yourself, do you define it as an indulgence or constrict any pleasure within the confines of guilt? Is spending money a cycle of abundance and then crashing scarcity? If and when you are confident in your finances, do you give any of it away?

Wealth is not about the size of our bank account, but a state of consciousness. The Hebrew prophet Isaiah affirmed this in his statement, "The desert shall rejoice and blossom as the rose." Even in a state of dearth—whether that is within our finances, a relationship, or work—living merrily as if amidst roses creates space for welcoming in abundance.

This framework allows for the release of old patterns of scarcity, where we expect to never have enough, feel undeserving of prosperity or success, and turn a blind eye toward the abundance we already have. Our job here then is not to beg and plead for financial abundance, but to provide thanks as if we already have it.

Yet sometimes our desires appear to be denied. That is when we can replace our old, habitual programming around money with a new code for prosperity—like a mantra of affirmation that a state of wealth is available to all. Sometimes the end-product of our desires is beyond what we have envisioned, in a different package, received at the eleventh hour. Establish faith that the harvest will come when you stop waiting impatiently, surrender, and lift your eyes.

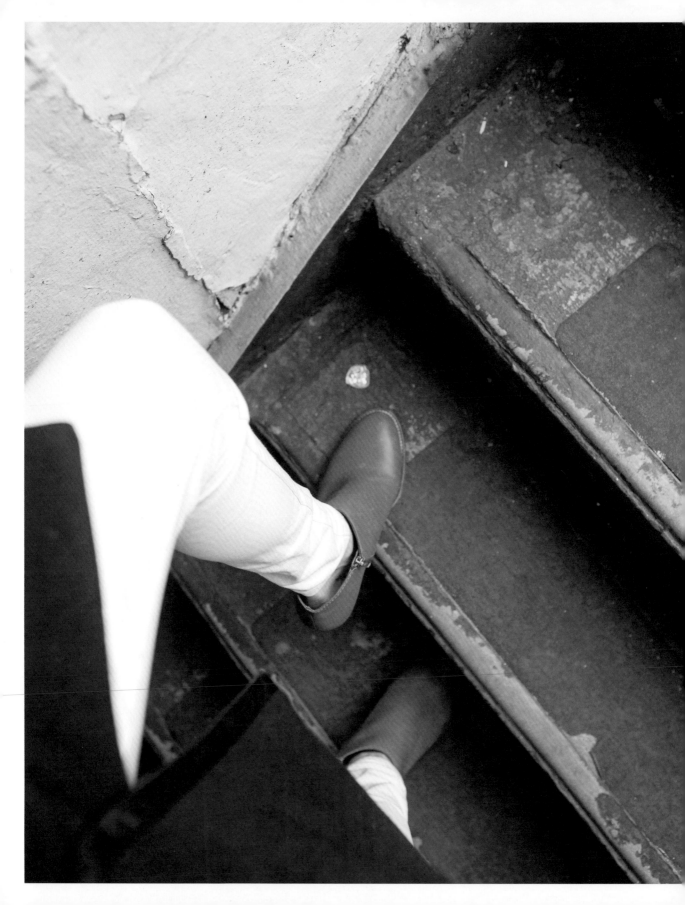

MARCHING INTO DISAPPOINTMENT

"We must surrender our hopes and expectations, as well as our fears, and march directly into disappointment, work with disappointment, go into it, and make it our way of life, which is a very hard thing to do."

— CHÖGYAM TRUNGPA

Gripped by desire, we often clench onto wishful outcomes. Yet the subconscious has had enough experience with disappointment to arm itself against it. But when we shield our vision away from facing disappointment and focus solely on the hoped-for outcome, we are doing ourselves a disservice.

To truly manifest is to attract what will universally serve us most highly, whether that is what we have envisioned or not. When we speak our desires to the Universe, we must do so with open arms that embrace both the desired outcome and the disappointment.

It is only when we open up this way—when we are sharp and direct with our wishes—that we flow into the reality of the situations we face. We become a sanctuary for ourselves rather than a container for various outcomes. May we be containers for ourselves and hold space for all that can enter into our lives.

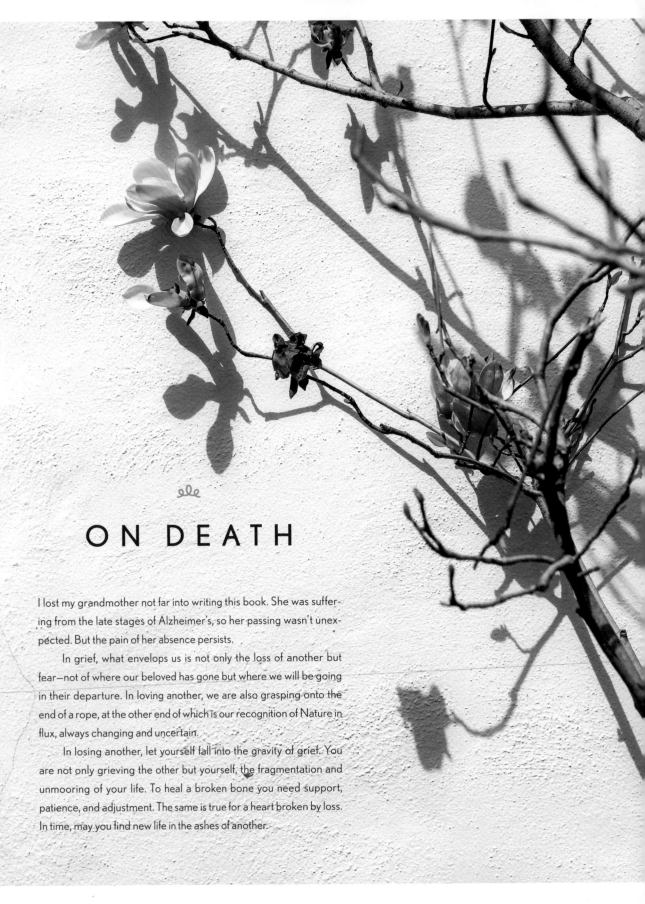

ON DEATH

I lost my grandmother not far into writing this book. She was suffering from the late stages of Alzheimer's, so her passing wasn't unexpected. But the pain of her absence persists.

In grief, what envelops us is not only the loss of another but fear—not of where our beloved has gone but where we will be going in their departure. In loving another, we are also grasping onto the end of a rope, at the other end of which is our recognition of Nature in flux, always changing and uncertain.

In losing another, let yourself fall into the gravity of grief. You are not only grieving the other but yourself, the fragmentation and unmooring of your life. To heal a broken bone you need support, patience, and adjustment. The same is true for a heart broken by loss. In time, may you find new life in the ashes of another.

And through the black bitter waters of the night
A cold velvet dip into your absence
The distant laugh from a Spring window, ajar
Drifting my sail away
A compass for the one to depart after the departed
and will it point toward you?
—trailing
Lost in the sea, may I burn to flames
on your stove, in your half-lived room
Into ashen memories
No longer to be of the soil, the flower, a daring sun
But to wither into dust
And be ash to your ashes
In a jar, preserved
Until
Strewn across a wasteland
And even then
will we meet in terra firma
to become soot to soften the land
And sprout into a flower of
You
    And
Me.
And I

Of blood churned
Frothing over with life
Yet to bear
Thinking of death.
I'll live to live for you
are there
or here
To face death now or later,
in the next deal
But may we raise a negotiation
to the arrangement of funerals
Across the seas
Perhaps by the time of my death.
And when will I be released from my prison?
Like the whimper of an avalanche over a cliff
Something inside resounds:
soon.

———

The needle of grief
That pierces the skin
Strokes the vein of your memory still
Tugging my boat, anchored
In its yellowed light diverting the nightfall
Nailing stars to my fingertips
To pull on the sails of a morning

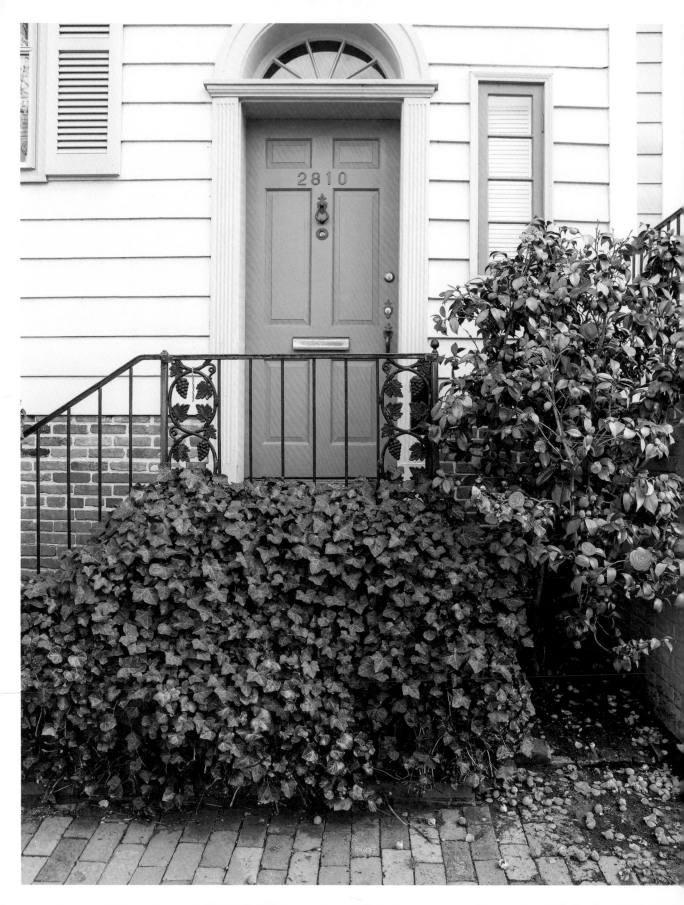

OPENING & CLOSING DOORS

How many times have you held the knob of a door in trepidation of what lay behind it? What door have you walked towards only to find your knees giving way at its steps? And do you remember the door from which you first stepped out of? We often find ourselves in fear of what we are about to embark upon, or contemplating choices in our past.

We might find ourselves behind that opened door, on the new path, having forgotten the places, choices, and the people who have made us who we are. Or we realize we are constantly looking back, thinking of our past life. Did you shut it behind you, is it locked? Do you check your pockets for the comfort of feeling the key? And sometimes we discover the door of our past unlatched, with only one foot in the present and the other ready to run to the comfort of what we left behind. We mindlessly walk toward that door opening to habits or people that do not serve us. But do not waste your time jumbling your keys to enter into the past. The door to our own true self will always hang slightly ajar to welcome in our maybe-one-day muddy feet in the chance of a storm pouring upon us.

Where is the door to your home? Have you misplaced it? Our personal version of home can be a physical place, or wherever our biological or chosen family is. It can be a state of mind, coming easily to some and less so for others. It may take years to find and define what home means, but it may happen in an epiphanic instant. I've found that this practice of closing doors behind us—once we've had time to feel, process, grieve each stage of life or relationship those doors represent—allows us to surrender into moving closer to feeling at home with ourselves.

In moments when we may feel insecure, we can be tempted to knock on the door of another's home. Yet they, too, have something stirring behind their door. Sometimes there are hearts who house us still but cannot open their doors to us; they may be unable to come home to themselves. We must be home in ourselves to welcome in others. Let this be a reminder that instead of shuffling for the key to his or her door when it pours, may we pat the key to our own in our heart-pocket. May we remember that door left ajar.

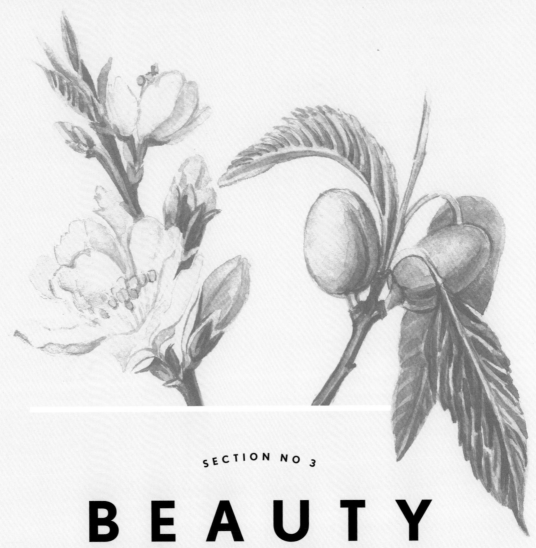

SECTION NO 3

BEAUTY BITES

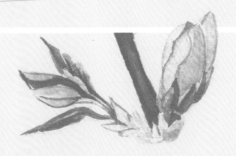

The recipes I offer you here are to

ELEVATE BEAUTY.

From the experiences they will cultivate in the kitchen, to the slow savoring of a first bite, they're here to sharpen your senses to the small pleasures of life. They are recipes with carefully curated ingredients that will tickle your palate and nourish your body. Here you will find recipes that feed the eyes and the body, sensitizing you to see eating as a multidimensional experience.

We're all learning, both supporting and challenging our long-held beliefs. It was only a few years ago that sugar was queen, low-carb was the craze, and fat was shunned. Now we know that sugar is the devil's breast milk and fat is phat.

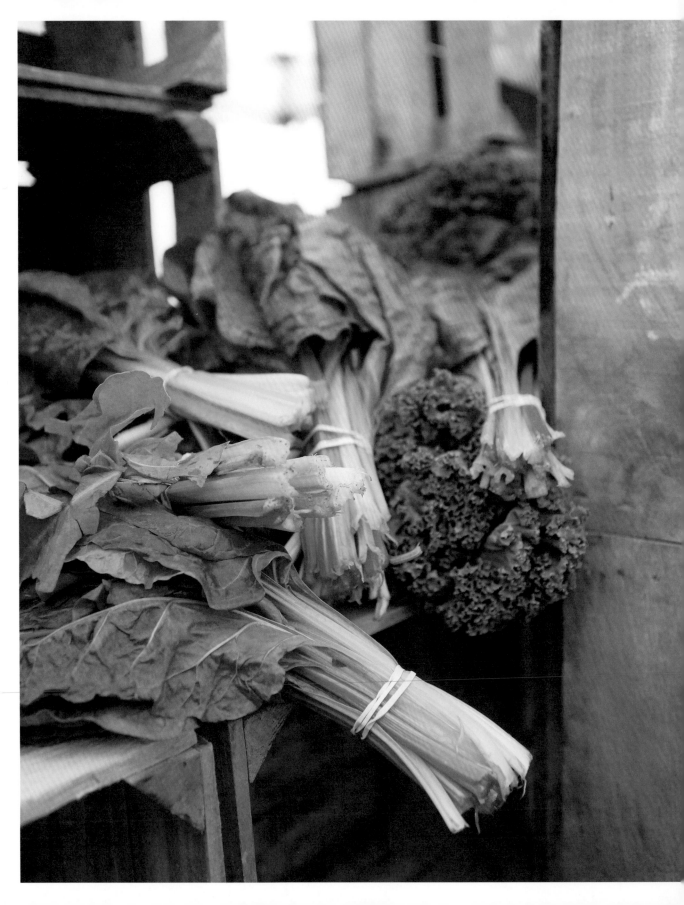

STOCKING YOUR KITCHEN

I advocate eating locally, organically, and seasonally as much as possible. Research proves these foods are higher in nutrition. For instance, organic dairy contains 62 percent more omega-3s than non-organic.[1] Various factors affect the nutritional quality of produce, namely the methods of picking, processing, and packaging. And even when the highest of grades are met for post-harvest management, foods grown further away lose most of their nutrients in the time it takes to get them to market. Spinach, for example, can lose as much as 90 percent of its vitamin C content in the first three days post harvest.[2] In addition to being healthier, local foods require only minimal mileage to get to market, which means they avoid the need for processing or machinery and minimize or even eliminate packaging. Buying local also supports the surrounding economy, especially the local farmers who prioritize taste over high yields, which is the opposite of what large corporate farms do.

While I encourage eating local, organic, and seasonal food, I'm also mindful of food deserts and the fact that many populations suffer from a crippling lack of access to this kind of nutritional bounty. As someone who studied medical anthropology, I am thoroughly aware of the broken food system and the ensuing obesity epidemic. That is a topic that deserves due justice outside of this book, but what food deserts connect to here is the current overconsumption of processed foods. Eating fresh and with the seasons, on the other hand, is an ancestral and sustainable practice. With modern technology comes the ability to eat a sweet peach in winter or dried Colombian gooseberries in Chicago, but there are drawbacks. Eating non-seasonally bends the rhythm of Nature, and often requires the use of pesticides, waxes, and other chemicals to grow or preserve foods.

Freshly harvested, in-season foods are at their peak in terms of antioxidant and vitamin content, but more importantly, they taste their best. Compare a juicy scarlet peach ripened by the summer sun versus one that matured in the crevices of a truck traveling through snow. Flavor promotes satiation, which means you need less food to feel full and satisfied. Furthermore, eating by the seasons creates a built-in rotation of foods and that prevents the body from experiencing stagnation, while also keeping food intolerances and allergies at bay.

This approach to eating is even in accordance with traditional Chinese and Ayurvedic medicine. Spring, for instance, is the season for detoxifying the liver in traditional Chinese medicine. Not surprisingly, it is also the season when bitter greens like dandelion are available to support this elimination process. In this, the seasons work synergistically with our bodies to enhance our health. To eat seasonally taps into the evolutionary wisdom of

Nature, and communicates biochemically with our bodies to optimize their function.

Since seasonal or local produce is not available everywhere—I should know having lived on the border of West Texas—I've devised a few shopping hacks. First, shop at the perimeter of the store where fresh produce is stocked. Opt for organic produce, if available, especially when buying apples and other heavily sprayed fruits—The Environmental Working Group's (EWG) Dirty Dozen Guide is a great resource for which crops are the most pesticide laden. Frozen produce is a cheap and sometimes healthier option as it's often flash-preserved at peak nutrition. For instance, frozen cherries can retain up to 88 percent of their original antioxidants.[3] Make sure frozen produce doesn't contain any additives or preservatives. Choose canned produce last and stick to cans free of bisphenol-A (BPA), a known carcinogen and endocrine disruptor.[4]

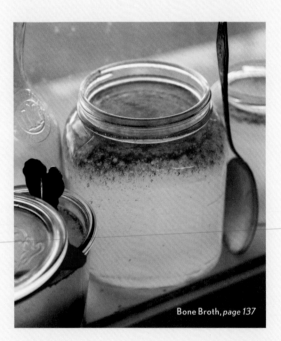

Bone Broth, *page 137*

There are also ways to prepare for when fresh, local produce isn't available and you need the nutrition or you're hungry for a particular fruit or vegetable. I grew up watching my grandmother pickle, ferment, and dry produce to use throughout the seasons and now I do this myself. Try making sauerkraut (page 178) or preserved lemons (page 179) to preserve seasonal nutrition and flavor.

Local, seasonal eating is also tied to sustainability. Produce grown locally and enjoyed seasonally is more sustainable, but certain foods, such as coffee, superfoods, and meats, may not be available in your region. We cannot cast a blind eye to the coffee farmers who pick beans by hand and are often grossly underpaid. For dried goods, including coffee, as well as tea and superfoods like chia or hemp seeds, look for fair-trade or Rainforest Alliance certifications. These signal a commitment to fair wages and environmental preservation.

For seafood and meat, I recommend consuming them only when they are humanely and sustainably raised. Monterey Bay Aquarium has a guide for sustainable seafood, most of which is wild or troll-caught. Easy options also include BPA-free canned wild salmon or sardines, half a serving of which contains 30 percent of your required daily calcium. Choose grass-fed and -finished meats and pasture-raised poultry, which are more nutrient dense. For example, grass-fed beef contains up to five times more omega-3s,[5] three times more of the antioxidant conjugated linoleic acid (CLA),[6] and higher concentrations of vitamins and minerals,[7] than grain-fed beef. Keep your consumption to a mindful amount, being conscious of the planet and making more room for plants on your plate.

For plant-based protein, opt for nuts, seeds, and seaweeds. I suggest avoiding or minimizing the consumption of grains and legumes, as these foods are high in nutrient-inhibiting and inflammatory phytic acid. This is especially the case for those with an autoimmune disorder, which you can read more about on page 13. Anthropologically speaking, grains were introduced to our diet later in our evolution and even then they were different, as they came from unadulterated crops. Crop yields were also much smaller, so grains were eaten infrequently and when they were consumed, it was in a fermented form, such as sourdough bread.

If and when you do eat grains or legumes, and even nuts or seeds, opt for organic as much as possible. Prepare them properly by soaking them in filtered water with a teaspoon of apple cider vinegar and a dash of sea salt to break down inhibitors. Certain grains, legumes, nuts, and seeds can also be sprouted to increase the bioavailability of their nutrients. Gently roasting nuts and seeds after soaking further decreases their enzyme inhibitors. Cooking grains and legumes with a piece of kombu accomplishes the same thing, plus it reduces flatulence which, let's face it, is the *real* cause for concern.

If you tolerate dairy, seek out raw, grass-fed goat or sheep's milk and stick to cultured varieties. Raw dairy has living probiotics, enzymes, and immunoglobulin antibodies that are destroyed through pasteurization, but more abundant in cultured cheeses, kefir, yogurt, butter, and cream.[8] Those who do not tolerate pasteurized dairy can often safely consume raw grass-fed sheep or goat's dairy products, which have easier-to-digest milk proteins and added enzymes. Choose only full-fat dairy, the cream of which synergistically decreases the likelihood of insulin spikes from lactose (milk sugar) and aids in the digestion of casein (milk protein).

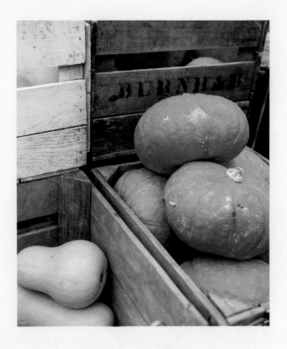

I use sweeteners sparingly but when I do I turn to raw coconut syrup, yacon syrup, or Manuka honey. The first two sweeteners are mineral-rich and low-glycemic, so they have a minimal impact on blood sugar levels, especially when used in small amounts. Although higher on the glycemic index, Manuka honey boasts a nutritional profile four times as high in B vitamins, amino acids, and minerals than other nutrient-dense raw honeys. This is called the Unique Manuka Factor (UMF) and the higher the factor number, the greater the nutrient density and the steeper the price. Manuka honey also contains increased levels of enzymes that create hydrogen peroxide, plus accompanying methylglyoxal and dihydroxyacetone, which give it anti-microbial, -fungal, and -viral properties.

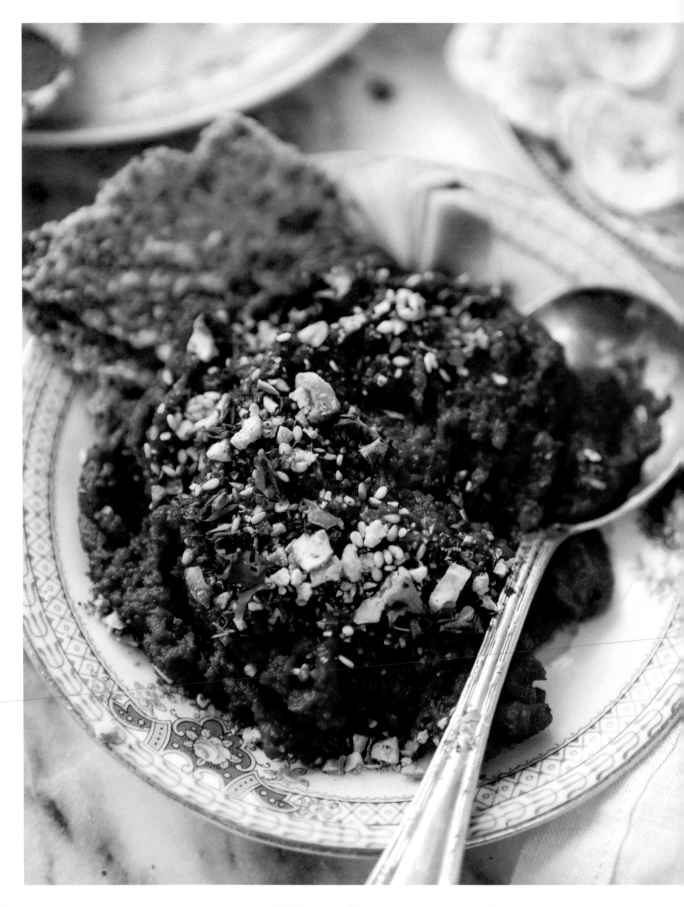

CHIPS & DIP

These chips and dip combinations make for satiating, healthful fat- and protein-packed snacks to nosh on while watching TV or to sustain your energy in the afternoon.

Herbed Crackers

MAKES 20 LARGE OR 40 SMALL CRACKERS

½ cup (70 g) nuts of your choice

¼ cup (302 g) pumpkin or sunflower seeds

2 tablespoons sesame seeds

1 tablespoon freshly ground flax seeds*

1 tablespoon chia seeds

½ cup (50 g) blanched almond flour

1 tablespoon cassava flour

½ teaspoon Himalayan pink salt

⅛ teaspoon each of garlic powder, dried rosemary, and dried thyme

1 tablespoon avocado oil or ghee

¼ cup (60 ml) filtered water

Preheat the oven to 325°F (160°C). In a high-speed blender or food processor, combine the nuts and seeds and grind into a flour. Add the almond and cassava flours, salt, and the herbs, and grind again to combine. Add the avocado oil and blend until combined then add the filtered water and blend again until a dough forms. Transfer the dough to a sheet of unbleached parchment paper and cover with a second sheet of parchment. Use a rolling pin to roll the dough into a thin rectangular sheet. Remove the top piece of parchment and transfer the bottom piece of parchment and the dough to a baking sheet. Bake until golden brown, about 20 minutes. Let cool on a wire rack before cutting into crackers or breaking them by hand. Store the crackers in an airtight glass container at room temperature for up to one week.

NOTE *Purchase flax seeds whole and grind them right before using, as they go rancid soon after grinding if not refrigerated or preserved properly.*

Flax Crackers

MAKES 10 LARGE OR 20 SMALL CRACKERS

1 cup (168 g) whole flax seeds*

2 tablespoons freshly ground chia seeds

¾ cup (180 ml) filtered water

2 teaspoons coconut aminos

½ teaspoon Himalayan pink salt

⅛ teaspoon each of garlic powder and dulse powder (optional)

Preheat the oven to 375°F (190°C) or set a dehydrator to 104°F (40°C). Line a baking sheet with unbleached parchment paper.

In a medium bowl, mix together the flax seeds and chia seeds. Add the filtered water, coconut aminos, and salt, along with the garlic powder and dulse powder, if using. Use a spatula to mix well then let stand, stirring regularly, until the seeds form a gel, about 15 minutes.

Spread a thin layer of the mixture onto the parchment-lined baking sheet and bake, flipping halfway through at 7 to 8 minutes, until golden brown and crispy, for about 15 minutes total baking time. If using a dehydrator, dehydrate, flipping halfway through, until dry to the touch, about 12 hours per side. Let cool on a wire rack before breaking into crackers. Store the crackers in an airtight glass container in the refrigerator for up 2 weeks.

NOTE *Purchase flax seeds whole and grind them right before using, as they go rancid soon after grinding if not refrigerated or preserved properly.*

Bean-Free Hummus

MAKES ABOUT 2 CUPS

Hummus and many similar creamy purées are made with legumes or dairy, which are inflammatory ingredients especially for those suffering from an autoimmune illness (page 13). This purée obtains its creaminess instead from root vegetables—either pumpkins or beets. If you are following a strict dietary autoimmune regime, opt for beet as the pumpkin's higher levels of lectins—plant proteins that can bind to cell membranes and cause tears in the gut—can aggravate autoimmune symptoms.

1½ cups (330 g) pumpkin or beet purée*
¼ cup (224 g) tahini
¼ cup (60 ml) lemon juice
2 cloves garlic, crushed and peeled
1 tablespoon extra-virgin olive oil
½ teaspoon Himalayan pink salt
¼ teaspoon each of ground white pepper and ground cumin

In a high-speed blender or food processor, combine the pumpkin or beet purée, tahini, lemon juice, garlic, olive oil, salt, white pepper, and cumin. Purée on medium-high until smooth. Serve the hummus immediately or store in an airtight glass container in the refrigerator for up to 2 weeks.

NOTE *You can buy canned pumpkin purée or make the beet purée. To make the beet purée, boil two large peeled beets in enough water to cover them in a saucepot. Boil until they're soft to the pierce of a knife, about twenty minutes. Remove from heat, pour out the hot water, and run cold water over them to cool. Cut them into quarters, place them in a high-speed blender, and blend until it reaches a smooth consistency.*

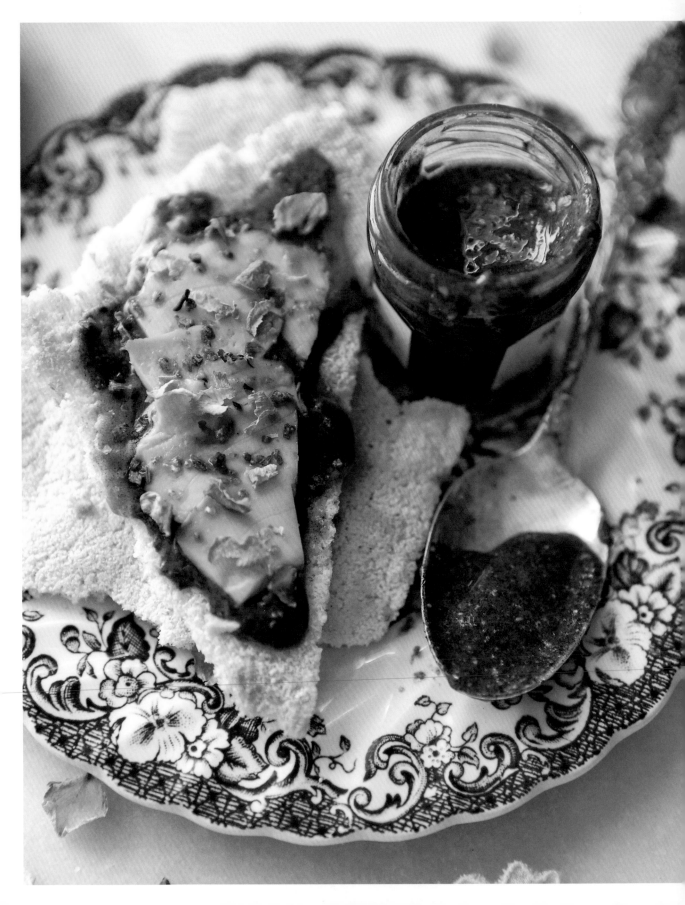

SIREN SPREAD

MAKES ABOUT ¾ CUPS

Siren Spread is an almond butter blend that developed out of my affinity for topping desserts with salt. When I make my own almond butter at home, I often add mineral-rich pink salt to make it more savory. While I enjoy plain almond butter, sweetening it slightly delivers a deeper hit to the palate, and satisfies more tastes. According to Ayurvedic medicine, our hunger cannot be completely satiated until all six tastes—astringent, sour, bitter, sweet, salty, and pungent—are fulfilled. This Siren Spread accomplishes this straight off the spoon, but it's also wonderful slathered on crispy apples or toast.

1 cup (140 g) raw almonds

¼ teaspoon apple cider vinegar

3 tablespoons coconut syrup,
    yacon syrup, or Manuka honey

1½ tablespoons spirulina

½ tablespoon coconut oil or ghee*

½ teaspoon Himalayan pink salt

Dashes of cinnamon and nutmeg
    (optional)

NOTE *Ghee will lend the spread a nuttier flavor.*

Prepare the almonds by soaking them overnight in enough water to cover them with a dash of salt and a ¼ teaspoon of apple cider vinegar. In the morning, drain, rinse, and dry them well.

Place the almonds in a high-speed blender or food processor and purée until smooth and buttery, about 1 minute. Add the coconut syrup, spirulina, coconut oil, and salt, along with the cinnamon and nutmeg, if using, and blend until fully combined. Store the spread in an airtight glass container in the refrigerator up to 2 months.

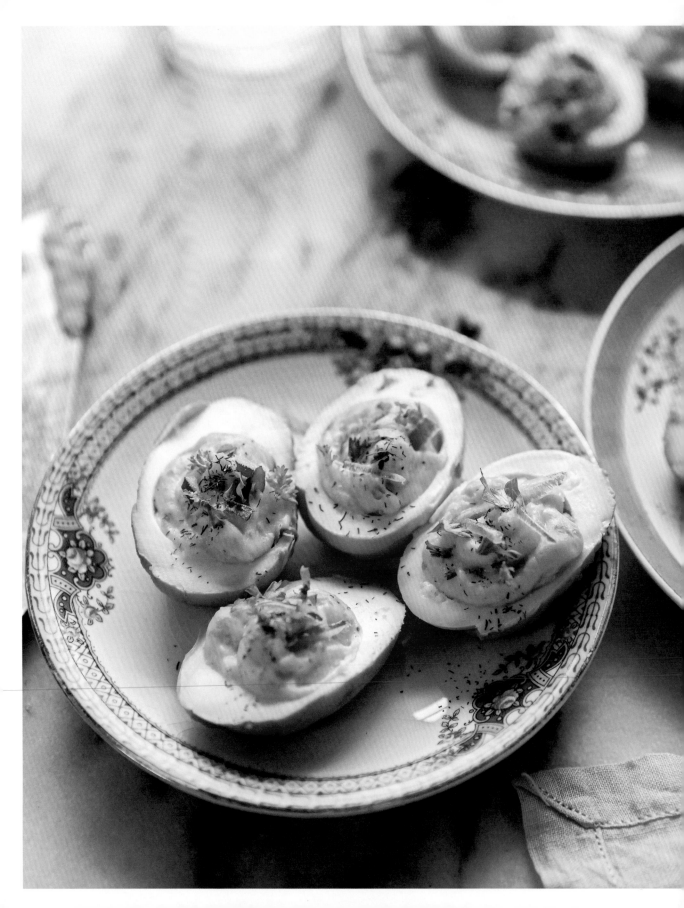

DEVILED EGGS

These deviled eggs get their incredible creaminess from the unexpected addition of Bean-Free Hummus made with pumpkin (page 129). This not only reduces the amount of mayonnaise, but also draws out the deep flavor notes of the cumin, as well as the sweetness of the pumpkin.

FOR THE MAYONNAISE

1 large, pasture-raised egg

1 tablespoon apple cider vinegar or freshly squeezed lemon juice

⅛ teaspoon dried rosemary

Pinch of sea salt

¾ cup (180 ml) avocado oil

FOR THE DEVILED EGGS

8 large, pasture-raised eggs

3 tablespoons Bean-Free Hummus (page 129)

2 tablespoons avocado-oil–based mayonnaise (see recipe above)*

1 tablespoon apple cider vinegar-based Dijon mustard

⅛ teaspoon ground cumin

Sea salt

Black pepper

Herb garnishes of your choice

MAKE THE MAYONNAISE Crack the egg into a large tall jar that's wide enough to accommodate an immersion blender—I use a ¾ L Weck jar. Add the apple cider vinegar, rosemary, and salt. Place the immersion blender inside the jar. With the immersion blender on low, very slowly drizzle the avocado oil into the jar and continue to blend until all the oil is added and the mayonnaise starts to thicken. Blend for 10 more seconds. Use the mayonnaise immediately or store in an air-tight glass container in the refrigerator for up to 2 weeks.

MAKE THE DEVILED EGGS Place the eggs in a medium pot, cover with cold water by 1 inch, and bring to a rolling boil over medium heat. Once the water is boiling, remove from the heat, cover, and let stand for 10 minutes. Transfer the eggs to a bowl filled with ice water and let stand for 5 minutes. Remove the eggs and gently roll on the counter to crack the shells. Peel the eggs then cut them in half and scoop the yolks into a medium bowl. Set the egg whites aside on a serving platter.

Add the hummus, mayonnaise, Dijon mustard, and cumin to the yolks and mash well to combine. Season to taste with salt and pepper. Place a spoonful of the egg yolk blend into each egg white. Top with garnishes of your choice, such as fresh or dried herbs. Refrigerate until ready to serve. Store the eggs in an airtight glass container in the refrigerator for up 1 day.

NOTE *You can find avocado-oil–based mayonnaise at most grocery stores or online health food shops. However, a homemade version will fare better with the quality of pasture-raised eggs and apple cider vinegar in lieu of grain- or beet-based vinegars used in store-bought mayonnaise. These vinegars can also aggravate yeast or bacterial overgrowth.*

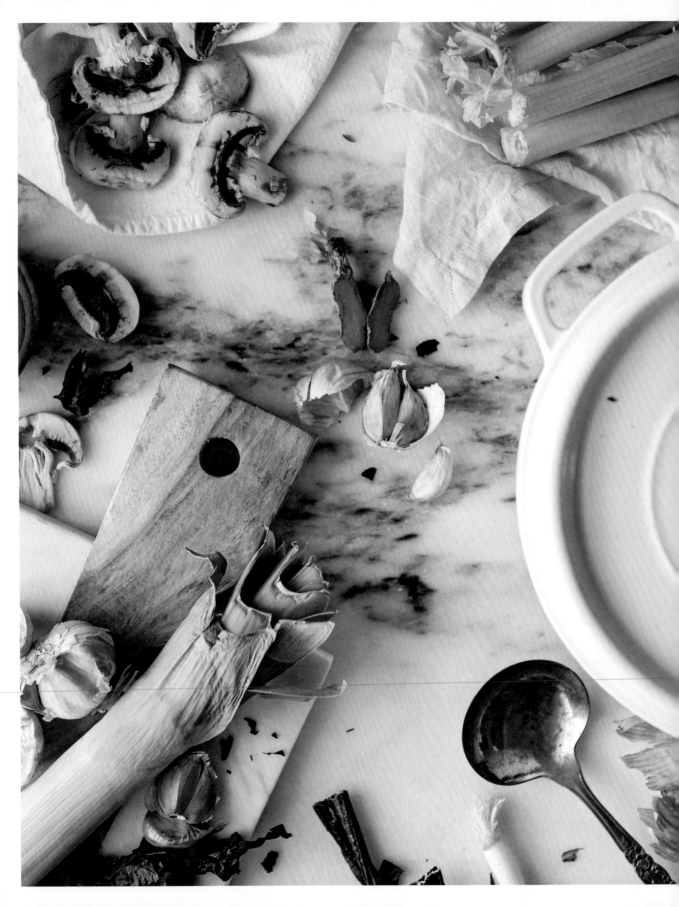

VEGAN MINERALIZING BROTH

MAKES 16 CUPS

A vegan option to rival bone broth, this nutrient-dense, plant-based recipe is full of minerals and vitamins synergistically combined with healthy fats to increase bioavailability. It's a forgiving recipe, so feel free to toss in vegetable scraps like broccoli stalks to reduce food waste.

Since the broth simmers for a lengthy period, I strongly suggest using organic produce to avoid any toxins like pesticides leaching into the soup. I also recommend thoroughly rinsing and scrubbing all the produce as an extra precaution. Organic vegetables also happen to have significantly higher concentrations of antioxidants and healthful compounds, such as 50 percent more anthocyanins and flavanols.[9] Anthocyanins give certain produce their vibrant hues and have anti-inflammatory, anti-cancer, and anti-viral properties, while flavanols prevent cell damage and consequently protect against cancer and other illnesses.

The broth's powerhouse ingredients include two types of seaweed, along with mushrooms and root vegetables. The wakame and kombu seaweed are sources of omega-3s, which many vegans are deficient in, along with electrolyte-balancing iodine, and minerals like magnesium, calcium, and iron. Shiitake mushrooms provide umami, imparting a meaty taste to the broth. They're also high in vitamin D from being dried by the sun, contain essential amino acids, and are prebiotic for intestinal health. Turmeric and ginger tint the broth with a sunny hue and provide anti-inflammatory properties. When the curcumin of the turmeric is combined with black pepper, its potency is increased sevenfold, up to 2,000 percent.[10] The coconut oil ties all the ingredients together, infusing a subtle sweetness and allowing fat-soluble vitamins like vitamin A, D, E, and K to be fully absorbed by the body.

Recipe Continues

2 tablespoons coconut oil

1 bunch celery, cut into chunks

2 carrots, unpeeled and cut into small chunks

1 yellow or red onion, cut into chunks

4 cloves garlic, halved

1 (3-inch / 7.5 cm) piece fresh organic turmeric, peeled and roughly chopped

1 (3-inch / 7.5 cm) piece fresh organic ginger, peeled and roughly chopped

2 cups (85 g) kale, stems removed and roughly chopped

1 Japanese or regular sweet potato, unpeeled and cut into chunks

½ cup (64 g) dried shiitake mushrooms (no need to soak) or 1 cup any fresh whole mushroom

¼ cup (5 g) fresh flat-leaf parsley, roughly chopped

1 (8-inch / 20 cm) piece kombu

Handful of dried wakame or dulse

1 dried bay leaf

½ tablespoon Himalayan pink salt

1 teaspoon black pepper

4 quarts (3.8 l) filtered water

In a large stockpot, heat the coconut oil over medium-low heat. Add the celery, carrots, onion, garlic, turmeric, and ginger and sauté until tender, about 10 to 15 minutes. Add the kale, sweet potato, mushrooms, parsley, kombu, wakame, bay leaf, salt, and pepper, along with the filtered water, and bring to a simmer. Reduce the heat to low, cover, and simmer about 2 hours. Carefully strain the broth. Serve the broth immediately or store in glass jars in the refrigerator for up to 5 days. The broth can also be poured into silicone ice cube trays and frozen as cubes for up to 6 months.

BONE BROTH

MAKES 6 QUARTS (5.7 LITERS)

Bone broth was one of the first animal-based foods I introduced to my diet after switching from being vegan. Boasting high levels of gut-healing and inflammation-taming gelatin, along with anti-aging collagen and mineralizing micronutrients, it also has an arsenal of properties to support longevity, without the toxicity of botox. And it has the added benefit of being injected naturally into the cells via a bowl and spoon. Bone broth is deeply nourishing for those with weak constitutions, poor digestion due to restrictive diets, or any kind of malnutrition, such as a vitamin deficiency.

I seek out local, pasture-raised meat from a butcher shop, which supports the surrounding economy and is now a rare experience with the expansion of grocery store meat aisles. If the bones have meat attached, don't worry—it will add extra flavor. Chicken feet are optional, but they add additional healing gelatin.

3 to 4 pounds (1.4 kg to 1.8 kg) organic, grass-fed oxtail and/ or beef thigh, neck, or knuckle bones

3 chicken feet (optional)

¼ cup (60 ml) raw, unpasteurized apple cider vinegar

8 quarts (7.6 l) filtered water

OPTIONAL VEGETABLES AND HERBS

3 organic yellow onions, thickly sliced

1 (2-inch / 5 cm) piece organic fresh young ginger root, with peel

1 (1-inch / 2.5 cm) piece organic whole fresh turmeric root, with peel

Sprig of fresh rosemary

Place the bones and chicken feet, if using, in a large stockpot. Add the apple cider vinegar, along with enough filtered water to just cover the bones. Let stand at least 30 minutes and up to 1 hour to leach the minerals out of the bones and into the broth. Add the vegetables and herbs of your choosing, along with any scraps you might have on hand and the rest of the filtered water, and bring to a boil. Reduce the heat to low and simmer at least 24 hours to ensure the maximum drawing out of nutrients from the bones. Ideally, the broth will simmer for 72 hours to ensure a dark, rich, and gelatinous broth. Let cool to room temperature. Store the broth in glass jars in the refrigerator for up to 5 days. Leftovers can be frozen into ice cubes, preferably in silicone trays for easy removal.

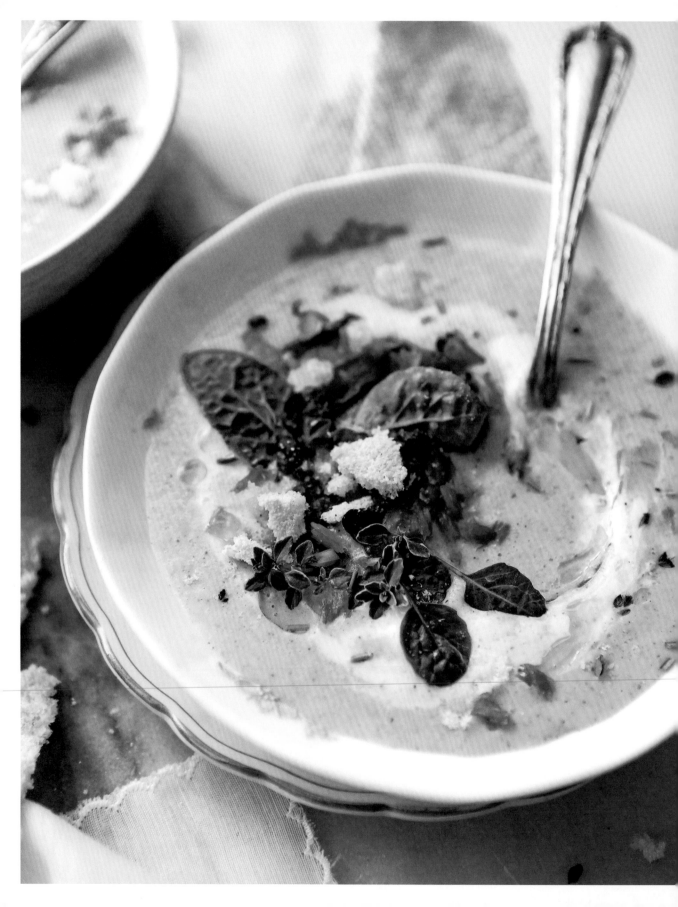

WILD MUSHROOM CHOWDER

MAKES 4 SERVINGS

This recipe is based on my chicken pot pie soup and was born out of the desire to accommodate a vegan dinner guest. The velvety base has a thick roux-like consistency, which it gets from cassava flour and a creamy cauliflower purée.

Cassava flour is an incredibly versatile one-to-one replacement for wheat flour. Plus, unlike refined flours or even potatoes, the cassava root it's derived from is low-glycemic, so it helps stabilize blood glucose levels. It's also rich in B vitamins, which provide energy, and saponins, which ease inflammation and balance gut flora.

FOR THE CAULIFLOWER CREAM

1 cup (100 g) cauliflower florets, steamed until soft

¾ cup (180 ml) almond milk or other dairy-free nut or seed milk

1 tablespoon coconut oil or ghee

¼ teaspoon Himalayan pink salt

¼ teaspoon black pepper

FOR THE MUSHROOM CHOWDER

2 tablespoons coconut oil or ghee

½ cup (60 g) chopped shiitake, oyster, or other wild mushrooms

½ teaspoon dried oregano

Salt and pepper, to taste

2 tablespoons cassava flour

3 cups (720 ml) organic vegetable broth (page 135 for vegan broth) or bone broth (page 137) if not vegan

½ medium yellow or white onion, cut into 2 quarters then cut into ¼-inch-thick (5 mm) slices

1 Japanese or Hanna sweet potato, cut into ½-inch (1.25 cm) cubes

1 stalk celery or broccoli, cut into ½-inch (1.25 cm) pieces

2 small carrots, diced

1 dried bay leaf

¼ cup (5 g) chopped fresh flat-leaf parsley or herb of your choice

MAKE THE CAULIFLOWER CREAM Place the soft steamed cauliflower, almond milk, coconut oil, salt, and pepper in a small pot and use an immersion blender to purée until creamy. Set aside.

MAKE THE MUSHROOM CHOWDER In a large pot, heat a tablespoon of the coconut oil over medium-high heat. Add the mushrooms, oregano, salt, and pepper and sauté until soft. Transfer to a plate and set aside.

In the same pot, heat the remaining 1 tablespoon coconut oil over medium-high heat. Add the cassava flour and toast, stirring, until it starts to brown, about 5 minutes. Slowly add the vegetable broth as you stir then add the onion, sweet potato, celery, carrots, and bay leaf. Reduce the heat to medium-low, cover, and cook until the vegetables are tender, about 15 minutes. Add the cauliflower cream and the cooked mushrooms, stir, and cook for another 5 minutes. Sprinkle with the parsley and serve!

NOTE *The chowder pictured here (opposite) is garnished with fresh oregano, micro greens, sautéed mushrooms, olive oil, dehydrated yucca root, and coconut yogurt (see page 179).*

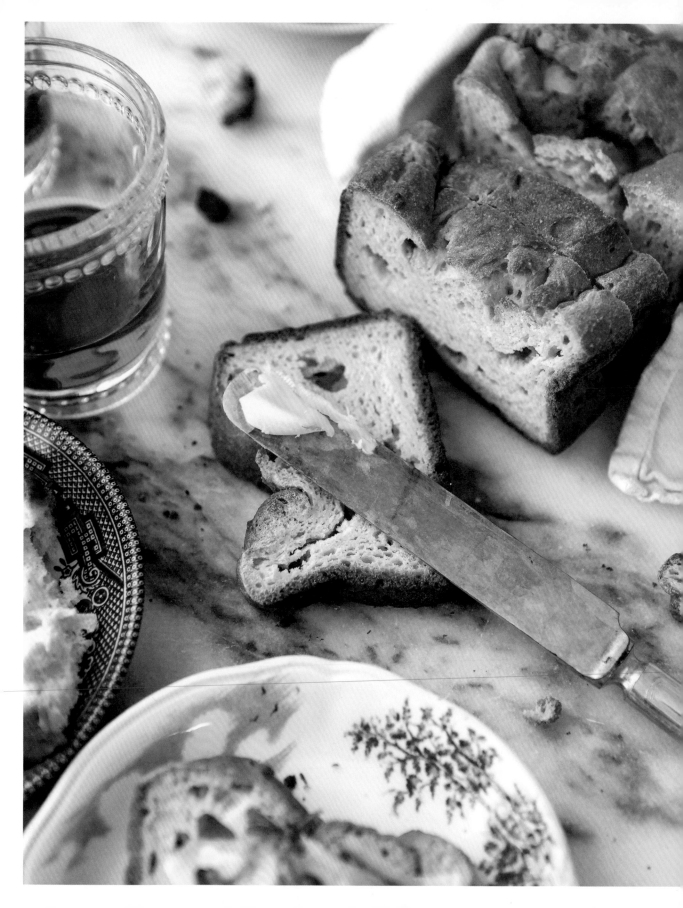

GRAIN-FREE SOURDOUGH HERB LOAF

MAKES 1 (9 X 5-INCH / 23 X 13 CM) LOAF

Making sourdough bread is an ancient practice that was devised not just to create a tangy flavor, but also to make grain-based breads more digestible. Grains have significantly high levels of antinutrients, phytic acid, and lectins. These compounds bind to and chelate vital nutrients, and inhibit the release of enzymes necessary for digestion, such as pepsin for proteins and amylase for carbohydrates. As a result, the body absorbs less of the available vitamins and minerals and the few it does obtain, it processes with difficulty due to lack of proper stomach acid function.

This sourdough bread is made with a base of nuts or seeds, which contain lower levels of phytic acid that are even further reduced by overnight soaking. Cassava flour, which comes from a tuber, is a one-to-one replacement for white flour, and gives the bread more substantial texture and flavor. The brine adds extra probiotics to make this bread even easier to break down and digest.

Eat the loaf spread with ghee and jam (page 161), or use it in stuffing for the holiday season.

2 cups (300 g) raw nut or seed of your choice

Filtered water, for soaking and rinsing

1 teaspoon Himalayan pink salt, plus a pinch for soaking

½ cup (120 ml) nut milk of your choice or filtered water

2 tablespoons brine from fermented vegetables, such as sauerkraut (page 178) or kombucha (page 174)

Coconut oil, for greasing

¾ cup (78 g) freshly ground flax seeds

¾ cup (90 g) cassava flour

1 tablespoon dried rosemary, lavender, thyme, or herb of your choice

½ teaspoon baking soda

2 large, pasture-raised eggs

3 tablespoons ghee, coconut oil, or avocado oil

In a large bowl, combine the nuts or seeds with enough filtered water to cover, add the pinch of salt, and soak overnight.

Drain and rinse the soaked nuts or seeds with fresh filtered water then drain again and place in a high-speed blender or food processor. Add the nut milk and brine and pulse a few times then purée on medium-high speed until smooth, about 2 minutes. Pour into a large non-reactive (glass, stainless steel, or ceramic) bowl, cover with a clean cloth, and place in a warm area away from direct sunlight—inside the oven with the light on works well if your home tends to be cool. Leave the nut mixture to ferment overnight.

When at least 24 hours have passed and the mixture smells tangy, preheat the oven to 350°F (180°C) and lightly grease a small 9 x 5-inch (23 x 13 cm) bread loaf pan with coconut oil.

Add the flax seeds, cassava flour, dried herbs, baking soda, and the remaining 1 teaspoon salt to the fermented mixture and mix to combine. In a small bowl, beat together the eggs and ghee with an electric mixer. Add to the bread mixture and whisk with the mixer until smooth. Pour the batter into the prepared bread pan and bake until a toothpick inserted in the center comes out clean, about 45 minutes. Let cool completely before serving. Store the bread in an airtight container in the refrigerator for up to 1 week or the freezer for up to 2 months.

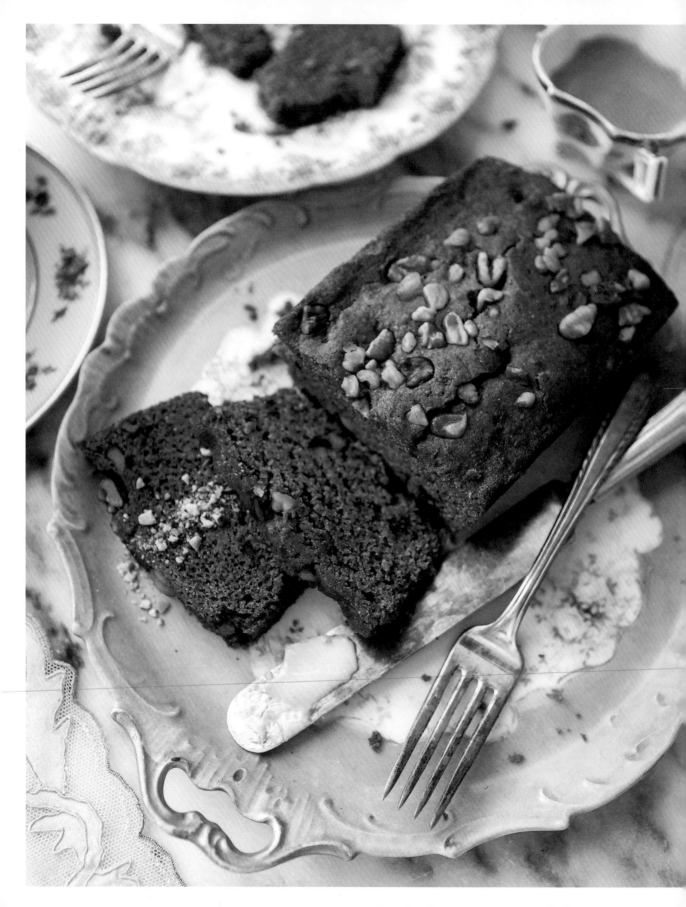

ALMOND BUTTER–MACA BREAD

MAKES 1 (8 X 4-INCH / 20 X 10 CM) LOAF OR 12 MUFFINS

I love breads and buns, but it's a difficult passion to bite into with celiac disease. My family doesn't make it any easier: My mother believes a meal isn't complete without bread and my grandfather constructs "bread sandwiches"—a torn piece of bread topped with salt and another piece of bread—ad infinitum.

When I switched to a grain-free diet, I longed for even the crumbs of store-bought gluten-free yet grain-based bread. This Almond Butter-Maca Bread was one of my first grain-free baked creations. With its light texture and deep flavor that's reminiscent of butterscotch, it's an ode to my bread-loving family.

Coconut oil, for greasing

1 cup (227 g) raw almond butter

4 large, pasture-raised eggs

1 tablespoon maca powder*

1 tablespoon ground cinnamon

1 teaspoon baking soda

1 teaspoon vanilla powder

1 teaspoon liquid stevia

Crushed nuts of your choice for topping (optional)

Preheat the oven to 325°F (160°C). Grease an 8 x 4-inch (20 x 10 cm) loaf pan with coconut oil and line it with unbleached parchment paper. Or line a 12-cup muffin tin with paper liners. (I prefer silicone cups to reduce waste. If you're using paper, opt for unbleached, compostable cups.)

In a large bowl, combine the almond butter and eggs and mix until creamy. Add the maca powder, cinnamon, baking soda, vanilla powder, and liquid stevia and mix until well combined. Pour the mixture into the prepared loaf pan or divide it among the muffin cups. Top with the nuts, if using, and bake until a toothpick or fork inserted in the middle comes out clean, about 25 minutes for the loaf and 10 to 12 minutes for the muffins. The bread is done when you can press your finger into it and it springs back. Let cool on a rack before serving.

Store the bread in an airtight glass container in the refrigerator for up to 1 week. You can wrap the bread in thin, breathable cloth to absorb any excess moisture that may collect in the container once refrigerated.

NOTE *If you have a sensitive stomach, I recommend gelatinized maca powder over the raw version. The processing of the former, along with the removal of the starch, makes it more digestible and bioavailable. Heating the root also activates certain metabolites and nutrients that would otherwise be dormant. It takes 9 pounds (4 kg) of raw maca powder to produce 2 ¼ pounds (1 kg) of the gelatinized version, making it an even more concentrated source of nutrients. However, the heat does alter the enzymes and some nutrients that are preserved in the raw version, including anti-cancerous and thyroid-balancing compounds.*[11]

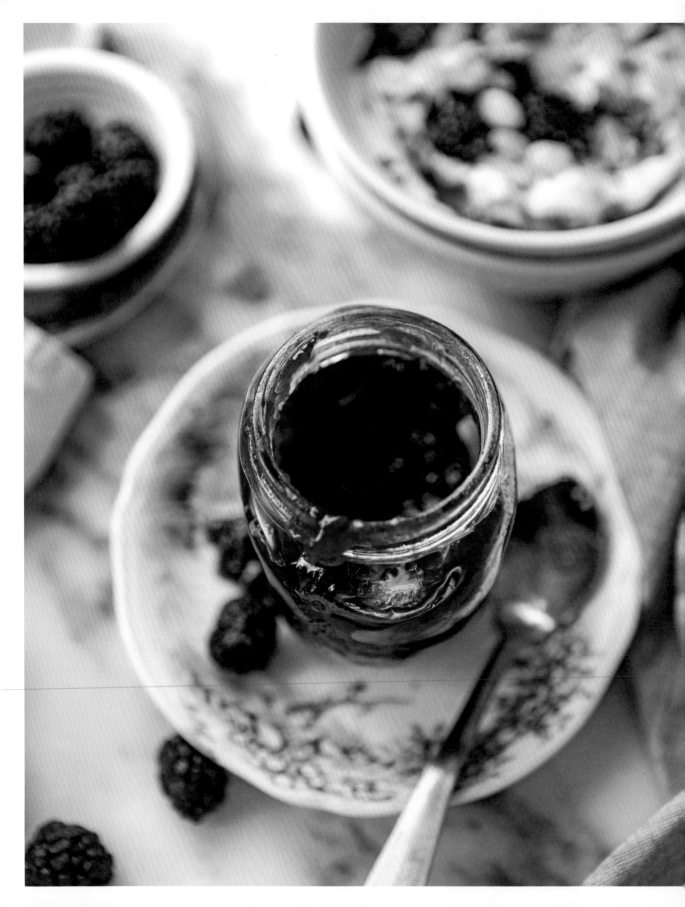

SPICED JAM

MAKES ABOUT 4 CUPS

My fondest memories of growing up in Turkey are dotted with baskets, bags, and hands full of fresh fruit. Every summer, my mother gathered local strawberries that were as small as a quarter but far sweeter than their mighty-sized cousins that I later eyed at grocery stores in the United States. Whenever I think of jam, I have a Proustian recall of the honeyed, ripe fragrance of her strawberry jam, so potent it even enveloped rooms behind closed doors.

Not surprisingly, when I gave up refined sugars, I didn't lose my craving for jam. I created this version not just to satisfy my palate, but to honor the fruits of my motherland. I make it on the eve of autumn, when fruits native to Turkey, including quince, figs, apricots, and persimmons are in full burst. My grandmother, who helped raise me, used to grow some of these in her garden, so I savor it in gratitude for her as well.

This is a very adaptable jam. You can use multiple fruits, as long as the total amount equals what's specified in the recipe. I'm partial to pure fig, as well as straight quince, or persimmon. Very ripe persimmon already has a jelly-like consistency, rendering the jam a texture reminiscent of marmalade, whereas quince makes for a much chunkier jam.

Jessica Koslow, a jam connoisseur and the genius behind Los Angeles's SQIRL restaurant, suggests using a copper pot to make jam—the copper allows for better temperature control.

2 ½ pounds (1.1 kg) fruit of your choice, cut into penny-size pieces (about 6 cups total)

2 cups (460 g) coconut sugar or erythritol*

2 lemons

2 cinnamon sticks

Dashes of nutmeg, allspice, dried rosemary, and Himalayan pink salt, added immediately once jam is done

2 (16-ounce) jars or one (24-ounce) jar

NOTE *Erythritol works perfectly well in this recipe, but coconut sugar gives the jam a deeper caramel flavor.*

Place the fruit in a large, preferably copper, pot and add the coconut sugar. Juice the lemons into the pot then wrap the rinds, along with the cinnamon sticks, into a piece of cheesecloth and secure with cotton twine. Add the lemon-cinnamon bundle to the pot and bring to a boil over high heat. Once the mixture starts to boil, push the fruit around from the sides of the pot into the center without scooping it. Continue to boil the jam as you continue pushing the jam, about 15 minutes. To test the jam, spoon a small dollop onto a plate and freeze for 3 minutes. Run a finger through the middle of the jam. If the line is clean, the jam is done.

While the jam is boiling away, sterilize your jars. Boil a stockpot of water, carefully add the jars and lids, and turn off the heat to let them sit.

Once the jam is done, add the nutmeg, allspice, rosemary, and Himalayan pink salt. Put on kitchen gloves and use tongs to carefully remove the sterilized jars and lids from the boiling water, gently shaking off any excess water. Spoon the jam into the jars, screw the lids on tight, and let stand on the counter until completely cool. Once opened, store the jam in the refrigerator for up to 1 month.

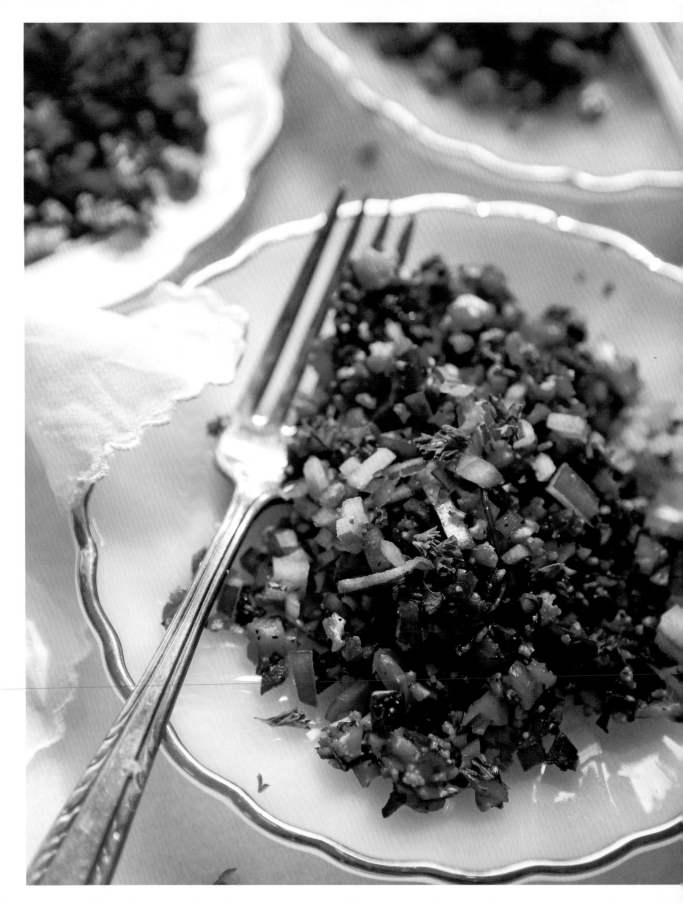

SWEET & SPICED CAULIFLOWER TABBOULEH

MAKES 6 SERVINGS

This recipe is influenced by *Kısır*, a cold Turkish mezze that's similar to tabbouleh and prepared with finely ground bulgur, parsley, and tomato paste. As a child, I had an always-realized fear of no leftovers, so whenever my mother made this special dish for guests, I'd request she set aside a couple servings just for me. Due to my autoimmunity, all of Kısır's main ingredients—except the parsley—are now off limits, so I created a modified version that's also more nutritious. For the base I use riced cauliflower and in place of tomato paste, my tabbouleh is sweetened with dried fruit, a staple of Mediterranean and Middle Eastern cuisines, plus carrots and orange juice for brightness.

1 small (9 ounces / 270 g) head cauliflower

¾ cup (40 g) finely shredded carrots or beets

½ red onion, finely diced

½ bunch fresh flat-leaf parsley, finely chopped

¼ cup (40 g) raisins or finely chopped dates

Juice of 1 orange

Juice of 1 lemon

2 tablespoons extra-virgin olive oil

¼ teaspoon ground cumin

Sea salt

Black pepper

Cut the cauliflower into quarters, remove the core, and place in a high-speed blender or food processor. Blend until the cauliflower is fine-grained like rice. Transfer to a large bowl, add the carrots, red onion, parsley, raisins, orange and lemon juice, olive oil, and cumin and toss well to blend. Season to taste with salt and pepper and serve immediately.

Store the tabbouleh in an airtight glass container in the refrigerator for up to 2 days—it will release extra juices.

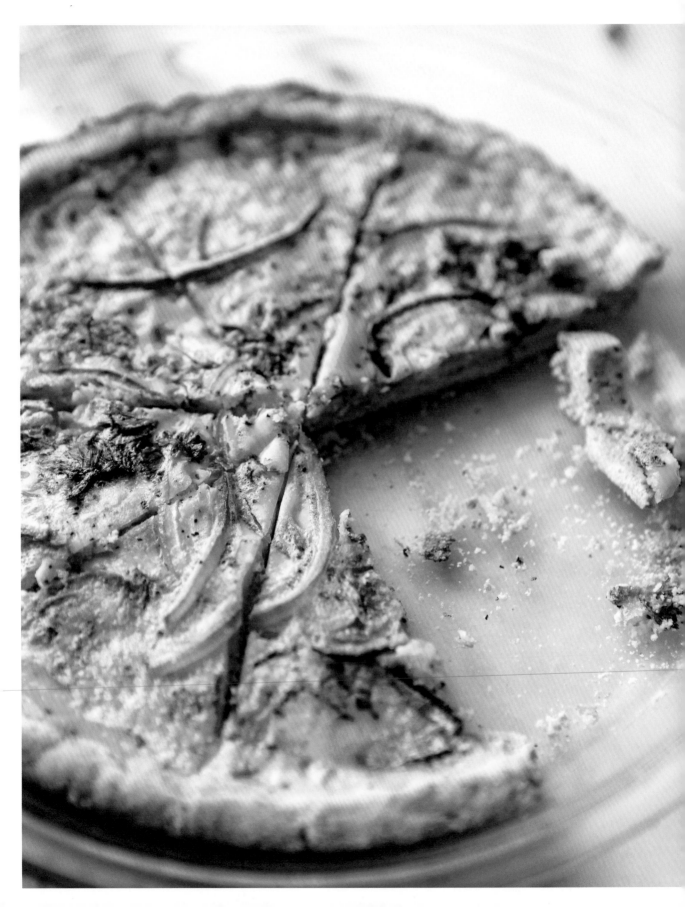

FARMHOUSE QUICHE

MAKES 10 SERVINGS

Quiche is one of the most elegant dishes yet is also one of the easiest to prepare, which is why it's perfect for entertaining. I also like to make it on late Sunday mornings when I want to feel a bit more refined, but I'm still in pajamas.

If you're short on time, you can chill the dough for just 30 minutes or skip the chilling step altogether. However, an overnight chill does make the crust especially light and flaky, so it's definitely worth the extra effort. The pastry does brown, but if you prefer a really crispy, golden crust, brush the dough with an egg wash, which is just a whisked egg yolk, before baking.

For the filling, I whisk a little water into the eggs to make them extra fluffy. Beyond that, the ingredients are simply suggestions. You can incorporate anything you'd like, from pasture-raised bacon and roasted sweet potatoes to salt-cured cod, which lends Spanish flair. I like to use Provençal herbs like thyme and rosemary, but lavender adds extra, unexpected flavor.

FOR THE CRUST

1½ cups (144 g) blanched almond flour

6 tablespoons (42 g) coconut flour

Pinch of Himalayan pink salt

Pinch of black pepper

2 tablespoons coconut oil or ghee, cold, plus additional for greasing

1 large, pasture-raised egg

1 tablespoon cold water

Dried herbs of your choice (optional)

FOR THE QUICHE

4 large, pasture-raised eggs

1 tablespoon water

1 handful fresh greens, such as baby spinach or arugula

6 pearl onions or 2 shallots, thinly sliced

Dried or thinly sliced fresh herbs of your choice

MAKE THE CRUST In a food processor or high-speed blender, combine the almond flour, coconut flour, salt, and pepper and pulse a few times to combine. Add the cold coconut oil and pulse until only a few little clumps remain.

In a small bowl, whisk the egg with the cold water. With the food processor or high-speed blender running, slowly add the egg mixture and continue processing until a ball of dough forms. Set aside.

Grease a 9-inch (23 cm) pie pan with coconut oil or ghee.

Arrange the dough on a piece of unbleached parchment paper and top with a second sheet of parchment. Use your hands to press the dough into a roughly 10-inch (25 cm) disc. Remove both sheets of parchment paper and place the dough in the prepared pie pan. Use your hands to gently press the dough to fit the bottom and up the sides of the pan. Refrigerate at least 30 minutes and preferably overnight.

MAKE THE QUICHE Preheat the oven to 350°F (180°C).

In a medium bowl, whisk together the eggs and the water. Add the greens, onions, and herbs and gently mix to incorporate. Pour the filling over the crust. Bake until the edges turn golden brown, about 20 minutes. Serve warm.

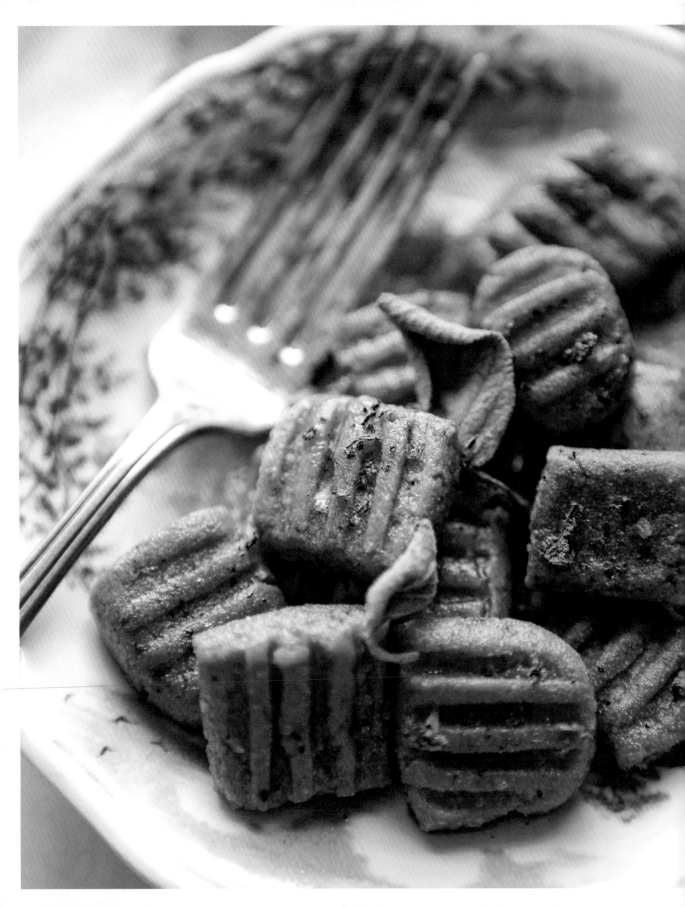

SWEET POTATO GNOCCHI

MAKES 2 GENEROUS SERVINGS

Gnocchi—or any variety of pasta—is either a dish you can enjoy in its traditional form or one you cannot eat due to allergies but that haunts you from the days when you could. As a grain-, dairy-, and nut-free alternative to classic gnocchi, this recipe offers comfort to both parties. You can even omit the egg yolk for a vegan version that's friendly to those with an egg allergy.

A decadent treat with a hint of sweetness on its own, this pasta is even more satisfying when served with a drizzle of extra-virgin olive oil and crispy, sautéed sage leaves.

28 ounces (840 g) Japanese, Hanna, or Korean sweet potatoes (about 2 medium)*

1 large, pasture-raised egg yolk (optional)

¼ teaspoon Himalayan pink salt

½ cup (60 g) cassava flour

NOTE *Do not use yams, as they're too moist.*

Preheat the oven to 400°F (200°C).

Roast the sweet potatoes without peeling until soft, about 30 minutes. Remove from the oven and let stand until cool to the touch but still warm, then peel.

In a medium bowl, mash the sweet potatoes with the egg yolk, if using, and the salt. Slowly add the cassava flour, 1 tablespoon at a time, until a dough forms—make sure the dough isn't too wet or too dry that it won't hold together. If dough is too wet, add flour. If too dry, add water along with a teaspoon of ghee. Form the dough into 4 (1-inch-thick / 2.5 cm) ropes then cut each rope into 2-inch-wide (5 cm) pieces.

Bring a stockpot of salted water to boil and cook the gnocchi in batches, adding them slowly to the boiling water and boiling just until they float to the surface, about 3 to 5 minutes per batch. Carefully scoop the gnocchi from the boiling water and transfer to a colander to drain. Alternatively, bake the gnocchi in a 325°F (160°C) oven until slightly golden brown, about 25 minutes. (Note that the baked version requires using an egg yolk in the dough.) Serve either version of the gnocchi as is or sauté in a pan with some ghee until browned for deeper flavor. Add dried herbs to your liking and serve immediately.

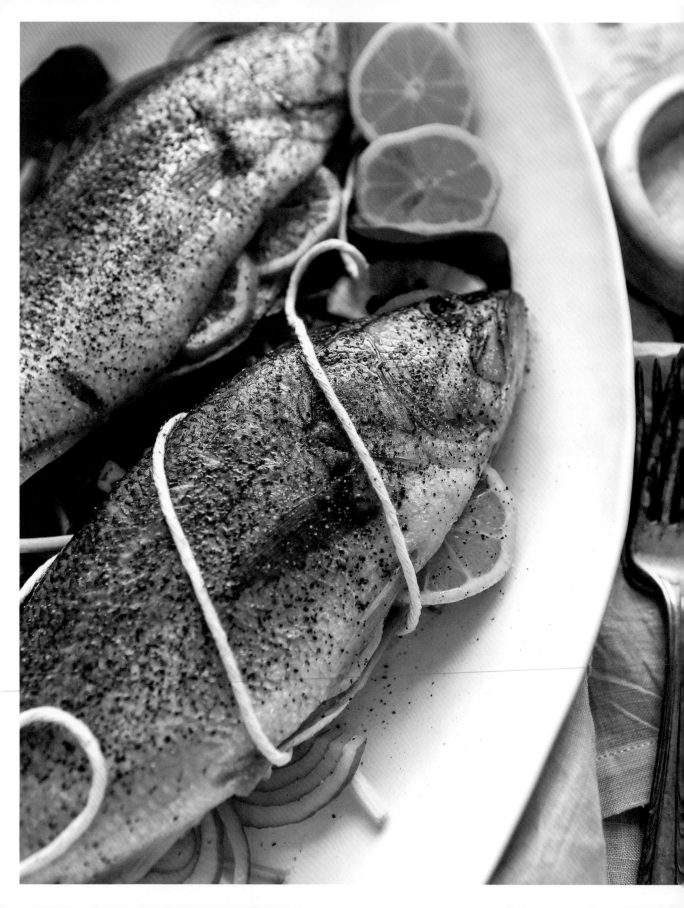

MEDITERRANEAN ROASTED WHOLE FISH

MAKES AS MANY SERVINGS AS NEEDED—1 FISH PER PERSON

If I have a signature dish, this is certainly it. With my Mediterranean roots and autoimmunity restrictions, cooking seafood was one of the first culinary skills I was determined to master. Both of my maternal grandparents hailed from small fishing ports near the Black Sea, so I considered my goal a dedication to their heritage and a way to give them a presence in my kitchen.

For my single mother, it's a way for us to connect. We make this dish, along with a simple salad, and gather around the table for what we call "Fish Fridays." It's also what I cooked after my first Thanksgiving with my husband's family, using it as a way to offer my gratitude for their open hearts and home.

The recipe below makes one serving, so it can be adjusted for however large your party may be. Roasting the fish on parchment-lined pieces of foil prevents sticking and makes cleanup easy.

1 (1 pound / 450 g) fresh, gutted whole branzino (also called European sea bass)

Himalayan pink salt

Black pepper

1 lemon

Preheat the oven to 425°F (220°C).

Rinse the fish under cold running water then set aside on a plate lined with a clean cloth.

Cut pieces of heavy-duty aluminum foil and unbleached parchment paper for each fish, making the pieces slightly larger than the size of the fish. Arrange the pieces of parchment paper on top of the pieces of foil and fold the edges over to secure them together. Generously salt and pepper both sides and the insides of each fish then place each fish on top of its own parchment-lined piece of foil. These will go directly in the oven as is, without a baking sheet.

Cut the lemon in half then cut a 1-inch-thick (2.5 cm) slice from the cut side of each half lemon.

Place 1 lemon slice inside the belly of each fish and another on top. Arrange the remaining lemon halves around the fish to roast alongside. Roast until the skin begins to brown slightly, about 20 minutes. To finish, broil the fish for 1 minute. Serve with the roasted lemon halves for squeezing over the fish.

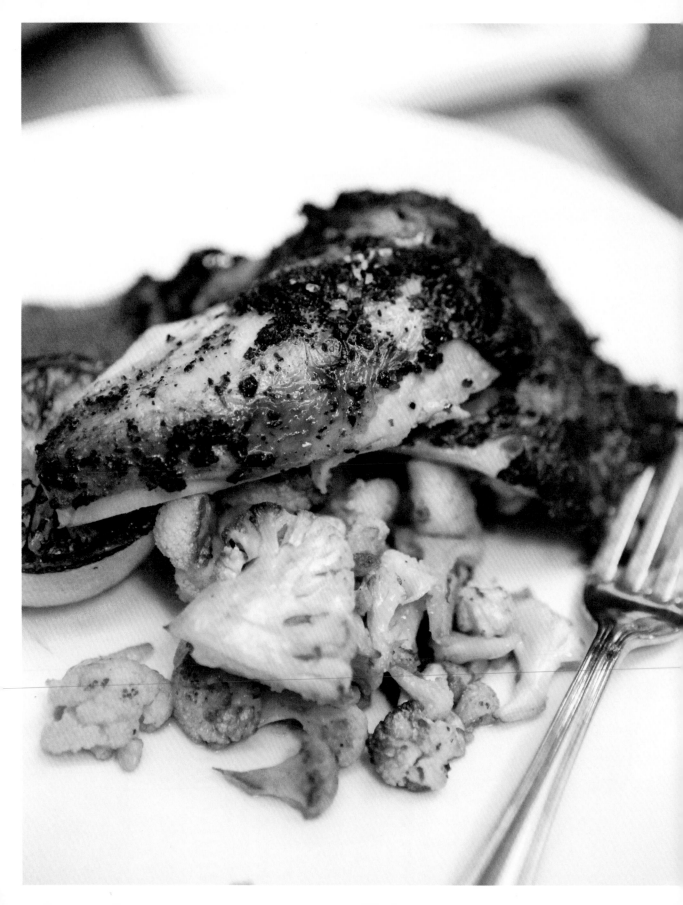

TRASH CHICKEN

MAKES 4 SERVINGS

This recipe satisfies a number of my culinary aspirations. First, I wanted to emulate charcoal-cooked Peruvian chicken, while simultaneously infusing the bird with Mediterranean flavor. I was also determined to find a better use for the leftovers than simply tossing the meat into a salad and putting the bones in the rubbish bin. In the end, I perfected the recipe, so that it makes three meals from just one whole chicken, including utilizing the bones that would otherwise have been trashed, hence the name. It's a true waste-free recipe!

After you roast and enjoy the chicken, any leftover meat, along with the spatch-cocked spine, can be made into a soup, using the chowder base on page 139 and replacing the mushrooms with chicken. The bones can be used in place of beef bones to make the bone broth on page 137.

½ tablespoon Himalayan pink salt

½ tablespoon dried oregano

1 teaspoon each of ground ginger, ground cumin, garlic powder, dried parsley, black pepper, and ground cinnamon

½ teaspoon ground cloves

1 whole (3 to 4 pound / 1.4 to 1.8 kg) pasture-raised chicken

2 tablespoons ghee or avocado oil

1 orange

In a small bowl, mix together the salt, oregano, ginger, cumin, garlic powder, parsley, pepper, cinnamon, and cloves.

Wash then pat dry the chicken inside and out. Place the chicken, breast-side down, on a large plate or rimmed baking sheet for easy cutting. Use heavy-duty kitchen scissors or shears to cut along each side of the vertebrae to remove it. Flip the bird and allow it to open like a butterfly by pushing down in the middle and on the sides. Rub 1 tablespoon of the ghee evenly over the entire chicken, making sure to get underneath the skin. Rub the seasoning mixture evenly over the entire chicken including underneath the skin. Zest half of the orange then juice it entirely. Pour the orange juice over the seasoned chicken along with the zest then refrigerate at least 2 hours and up to 48 hours. This allows the salt to fully tenderize the meat.

Preheat the oven to 425°F (220°C). Coat the bottom of a 12-inch (30 cm) cast iron skillet with the remaining 1 tablespoon ghee. Add the chicken, breast-side up, and roast until the skin is brown and sizzling, about 45 minutes. Transfer to a cutting board and let rest for 10 minutes before cutting and serving.

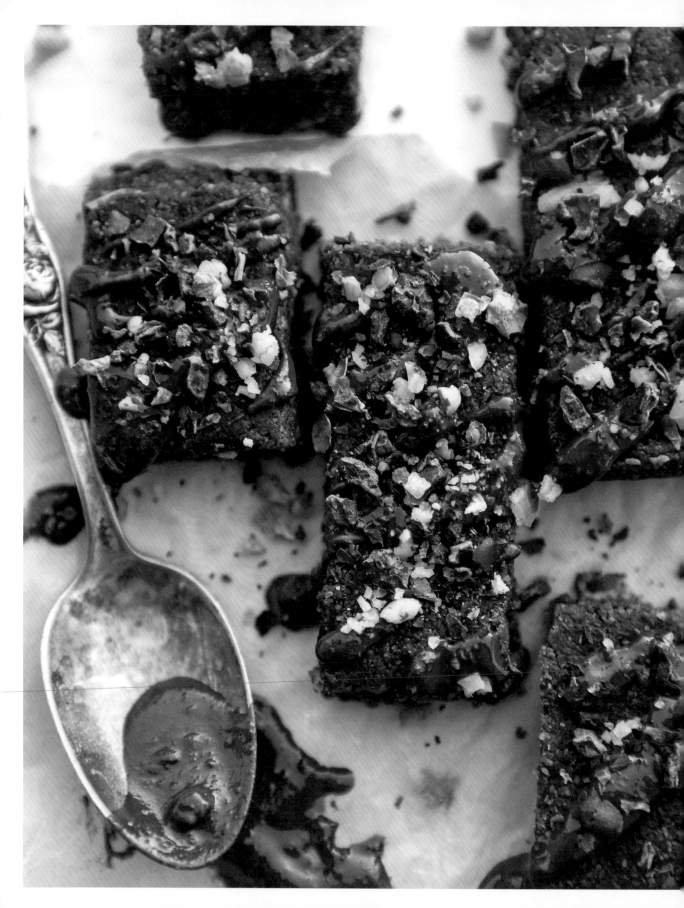

NUTTY CHOCOLATE HORMONE-BALANCING BARS

MAKES 10 BARS

Many women in the throes of their menstrual cycle crave chocolate, whether it's the body's way of signaling an iron or magnesium deficiency or simply a desire for comfort. Unfortunately, many of the chocolate bars on the market wreak havoc on hormones. They're often made with sugar, additives, soy, and dairy, all of which disrupt the delicate cycle of hormone production. Sugar-laden foods can eventually lead to insulin resistance in the body, taxing the thyroid and adrenal glands, which are responsible for balancing hormones.

These homemade bars satisfy chocolate cravings with pure cacao, which provides magnesium, zinc, iron, and calcium to replenish the essential minerals and energy that flow out during menstruation. They also contain coconut, a source of sustainable energy, and flax seeds, which are especially helpful for those who are estrogen-dominant. Elevated estrogen levels or an inability to flush out estrogen often leads to heavy bleeding, cramps, fluid retention, and weight gain, but flax seeds bind to excess estrogen receptors and block their uptake, allowing the body to eventually clear some of the excess. Flax also provides omega-3s, which have anti-inflammatory effects and promote healthy, glowing skin.

¾ cup (78 g) freshly ground flax seeds*

½ cup (90 g) chopped Medjool dates or dried mission figs

½ cup (46 g) desiccated coconut

¼ cup (32 g) pumpkin seeds

¼ cup (30 g) cacao nibs

¼ cup (25 g) raw cacao powder

2 tablespoons coconut oil

2 tablespoons nut or seed milk

1 tablespoon raw almond butter

1 tablespoon maca powder

½ teaspoon ground cinnamon

Dash of Himalayan pink salt

Crushed nuts of choice, cacao nibs, and flaked sea salt, for garnish

Line a 9 x 9-inch (23 cm) pan with unbleached parchment paper.

In a high-speed blender or food processor, combine the flax seeds, dates, coconut, pumpkin seeds, cacao nibs, cacao powder, coconut oil, nut milk, almond butter, maca powder, cinnamon, and salt. Blend on medium speed until a dough forms. Use your hands to press the dough evenly into the parchment-lined pan. Alternatively, roll the dough into balls and arrange on parchment-lined pan. Top with crushed nuts of choice, cacao nibs, and a dash of flaked sea salt. Refrigerate until firm, about 2 hours. Slice and serve! Store the bars in an airtight glass container in the refrigerator for up to 1 week.

NOTE *Purchase flax seeds whole and grind them right before using, as they go rancid soon after grinding if not refrigerated or preserved properly.*

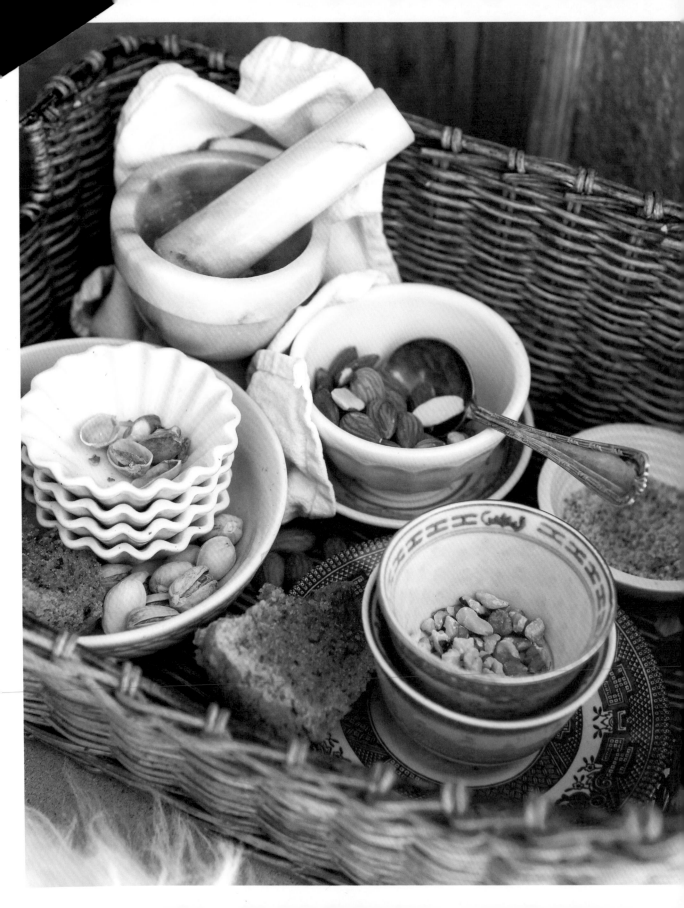

AYURVEDIC TRAIL MIX

MAKES ABOUT 2 CUPS

Nut and dried fruit trail mixes are wonderful to snack on, but depending on their quality, they can either elevate energy or wreak digestive havoc. Many conventional versions are roasted with vegetable oils, sugars, preservatives, and additives that cause a sluggish inflammatory response in the body.

This recipe follows the Ayurvedic recommendation of first soaking then gently dehydrating by toasting the nuts for optimum digestibility and absorption—this works for seeds too. Soaking reduces the amount of antinutrients present in nuts and seeds, while sautéeing provides the crunch we seek in trail mix. The ghee and spice mixture ensure that the digestive fire or *agni* is not compromised.

Fresh curry leaves are optional, but in addition to contributing flavor, they aid in liver detoxification. The lime juice added at the end rehydrates the mix for enhanced digestibility, and acts as a preservative.

¼ cup (35 g) each of almonds, walnuts, pine nuts, and macadamia nuts

Filtered water, for soaking and rinsing

Pinch of Himalayan pink salt

1 tablespoon ghee

1 sprig fresh curry leaves, whole (optional)

1 teaspoon garam masala

¼ teaspoon cumin seeds

¼ teaspoon ground cinnamon

¼ teaspoon vanilla powder

Pinch of Himalayan pink salt

¼ cup (45 g) each of chopped dates, raisins, and prunes

2 tablespoons lime juice

Chopped fresh cilantro or herb of your choice and freshly grated orange zest, for garnish

In a large bowl, combine the nuts with enough filtered water to cover, add the salt, and soak overnight.

Drain and rinse the soaked nuts with fresh filtered water then drain again.

In a large cast iron skillet, heat the ghee over medium-low heat. Add the curry leaves, if using, the garam masala, cumin, cinnamon, vanilla powder, and salt and toast for 30 seconds. Add the nuts and the dates, raisins, and prunes and sauté until golden brown, 10 to 15 minutes. Transfer to a plate and let cool. Add the lime juice and stir to blend. If enjoying immediately, garnish with cilantro and orange zest. If preparing ahead, store the cooled trail mix in an airtight glass container at room temperature for up to 1 week.

RAW COCONUT-ALMOND TARTLETS

with Lemon Curd & Raspberry-Rose Jam

MAKES 4 TARTLETS

There are a few recipes that jeopardize my self-control and these delectable tartlets might take the cake. I kid myself every time that I'll only have one then laugh halfway through a mouthful of my second. The bright, crisp notes of lemon and the easy sweetness of the raspberry make this a lighter dessert or an ideal brunch offering.

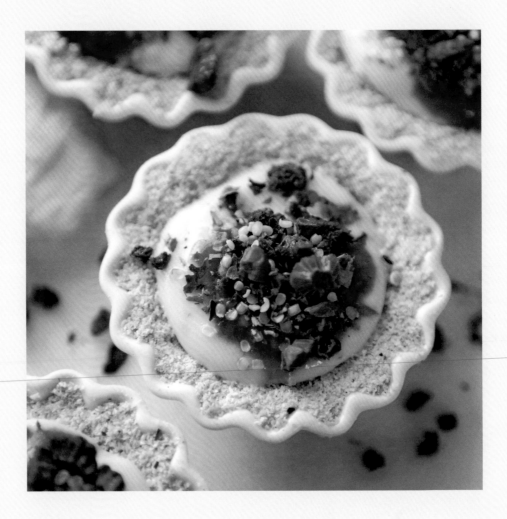

FOR THE CRUST

1½ cups (200 g) blanched almond
flour

1 cup (80 g) shredded
unsweetened coconut

1 tablespoon coconut oil

½ teaspoon liquid stevia

FOR THE LEMON CURD

3 large, pasture-raised eggs

3 tablespoons raw or Manuka
honey, maple syrup, or
coconut syrup

1 tablespoon freshly grated lemon
zest

Pinch of Himalayan pink salt

¼ cup (50 g) coconut oil

¼ cup plus 2 tablespoons (90 ml)
freshly squeezed lemon juice

FOR THE RASPBERRY-ROSE JAM

1 cup (125 g) fresh or frozen
raspberries

1 teaspoon freshly squeezed lemon
juice

1 tablespoon chia seeds

¼ teaspoon vanilla powder

¼ teaspoon rose water

1 teaspoon raw or Manuka honey,
maple syrup, or coconut syrup
(optional)

Dried organic rose petals, fresh
raspberries, or thin lemon
slices, for garnish

MAKE THE CRUST Place the almond flour, shredded coconut, coconut oil, and liquid stevia in a high-speed blender or food processor and blend until a dough forms. Divide the dough into 4 portions and press each portion into a 3-inch (7.5 cm) tart pan. Refrigerate for at least 1 hour while you make the fillings.

MAKE THE LEMON CURD In a non-reactive,* medium bowl, whisk together the eggs, sweetener of your choice, lemon zest, and salt. Pour the mixture, along with the coconut oil, into a small stainless steel saucepan and place over medium-low heat. Stir until the mixture is warm then add the lemon juice. Don't let the heat go above 170°F (77°C). Continue to cook the mixture, stirring constantly, until it thickens, 5 to 10 minutes. The curd is ready when you can run your finger through it on the back of a spoon and it leaves a clear trail.

Secure a piece of cheesecloth over a glass container and strain the curd through it. Let it cool completely then refrigerate the curd for at least 1 hour before filling the tarts. Store the lemon curd in an airtight glass container in the refrigerator for up to 1 week.

MAKE THE RASPBERRY-ROSE JAM In a small saucepan, bring the raspberries and lemon juice to a boil over medium heat, stirring and squishing the berries with the back of a spoon to release their juices. Once the raspberries have a syrupy consistency, remove from the heat, add the chia seeds, and stir until they plump up. Stir in the vanilla powder and rose water. If using a sweetener, add the maple syrup or coconut syrup now, but wait until the jam has cooled to room tempera-ture before adding the raw honey, as heat will kill the sensitive enzymes that are beneficial for digestion and mineral absorption. Let cool at room temperature. The jam will thicken in about 20 minutes. Store the jam in an airtight glass con-tainer in the refrigerator for up to 1 week.

ASSEMBLE THE TARTS Remove the chilled crusts from the refrigerator and place on a serving dish. Spoon the lemon curd into the crusts, filling them three-quarters of the way. Top the tarts with a small dollop of the raspberry-rose jam. Decorate to your heart's content with dried rose petals, fresh raspberries, or thin slices of lemon.

NOTE *Non-reactive materials include glass, stainless steel, and ceramic. For this step, avoid reactive utensils and pans such as aluminum, copper, iron, and steel.*

COURTESAN AU CHOCOLAT

MAKES 8 PASTRIES

These are inspired by the pastry treat called *choux au chocolat* in traditional French cuisine. A tower of these little cream puffs, in the pastel-hued world of Wes Anderson, is referred to as *courtesan au chocolat* in the director's *Grand Budapest Hotel*. Despite their charm, they're untouchable due to their lacing of gluten, refined sugar, and dairy. Here is my refined-sugar-free, dairy-free, and gluten-free adaptation, filled with chocolate ganache.

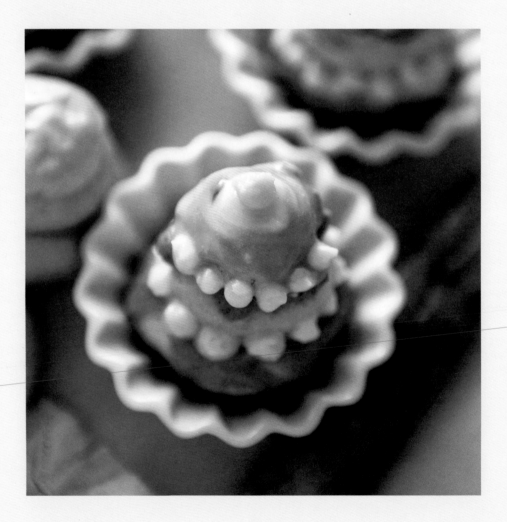

162

FOR THE CHOUX

¼ cup (60 ml) coconut milk

½ cup (100 g) coconut oil

6 tablespoons (85 g) arrowroot

2 large, pasture-raised eggs

Dash of Himalayan pink salt

Stevia (optional)

FOR THE CHOCOLATE GANACHE

¼ cup (57 g) coconut butter or manna, liquefied

1 tablespoon coconut milk

1 tablespoon raw cacao powder

Stevia (optional)

FOR THE COLORED ICING

2 tablespoons coconut butter or manna, liquefied

1 tablespoon coconut milk, plus more as needed

Stevia (optional)

Pink: 2 tablespoons pomegranate powder

Green: ¼ teaspoon chlorella

Purple: ½ teaspoon maqui berry powder or 2 mashed fresh blackberries

MAKE THE CHOUX Preheat the oven to 350°F (180°C). Line 3 baking sheets with unbleached parchment paper.

Bring the coconut milk and coconut oil to a boil in a small pot. Take the pot off the heat and quickly whisk in the arrowroot until fully incorporated. The mixture should look oily and gooey. Not to fret!

Place the goo-like mixture in a ceramic bowl, along with 1 egg, salt, and the stevia to taste, and blend with a electric mixer. Add the remaining egg and blend until creamy yet slightly sticky. Scoop the mixture into a piping bag fitted with a small tip. Pipe into 3 different size rounds onto prepared baking sheets: eight 1 tablespoon-size rounds onto a baking sheet, eight 1 teaspoon-size rounds onto a second baking sheet, and eight ½ teaspoon-size rounds onto a third baking sheet.

Bake all 3 sheets for 15 minutes then turn the oven off and allow the choux to sit inside for another 15 minutes until they're slightly golden brown. Watch the smaller choux closely, as they bake more quickly! Check and remove the small choux earlier if necessary. When done, transfer the choux to a wine rack to cool.

MAKE THE CHOCOLATE GANACHE In a small bowl, combine the coconut butter, coconut milk, cacao powder, and the stevia to taste and mix until creamy and ganache-like. Scoop the mixture into a piping bag fitted with a small tip.

Once the choux pastries are cool, use a small knife to make small incisions in the bottom of each pastry. Pipe ganache into the bottom of each choux.

MAKE THE COLORED ICING In a small bowl, combine the coconut butter, coconut milk, and stevia to taste and mix until it reaches the consistency of liquid icing. If the icing is too thick, gradually add more coconut milk. Divide the icing into separate bowls, add a different powder to each, and mix to create colored versions.

ASSEMBLE THE CHOUX Drizzle a colored icing over a large choux. Pipe a little ganache on the bottom of a medium choux and use it to "glue" the choux on top of the large one. Drizzle another colored icing over the medium choux. Pipe a little ganache on the bottom of a small choux and glue it to the medium choux. Finish by drizzling the last colored icing on top. Repeat with the remaining choux, ganache, and icing.

If you'd like to make the pearl decoration, slowly mix arrowroot into a spoonful of coconut butter until a slightly oily dough forms. Roll little pieces of dough into balls and place them on the choux.

Store the choux in an airtight glass container in the refrigerator for up to 5 days. Let it slightly reach room temperature by letting it sit on the counter before serving after refrigeration.

CREAMY CHOCOLATE HAZELNUT BARS

MAKES 12 BARS

These bars are inspired by Nutella, a childhood staple, and *pâte de noisettes*, which is more grown-up yet just as laden with oil and refined sugar. My version is decadent and richly textured enough to satisfy a sweet tooth with just a small slice; it's perfect for a snack or to serve après dinner. You must start these a day ahead, so there's time to soak the hazelnuts and cashews.

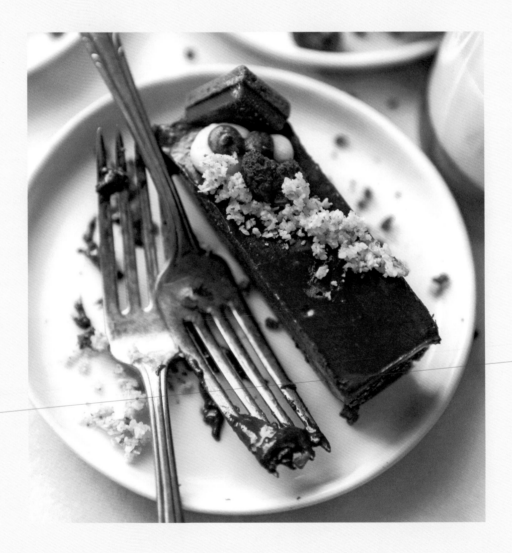

FOR THE CHOCOLATE-HAZELNUT BUTTER

⅔ cup (100 g) raw hazelnuts, without skin

Filtered water, for soaking and rinsing

Pinch of Himalayan pink salt

1 cup (118 g) raw cacao powder

⅓ cup (70 g) coconut oil

⅓ cup (113 g) raw or Manuka honey, maple syrup, or coconut syrup

FOR THE FUDGE LAYER

2 cups (300 g) raw cashews

⅓ cup (50 g) raw hazelnuts

Filtered water, for soaking and rinsing

⅓ cup (35 g) raw cacao powder

¼ cup (52 g) coconut oil

¼ cup (65 g) coconut butter or manna, liquified

¼ cup (85 g) maple or coconut syrup

½ teaspoon vanilla powder

¼ teaspoon Himalayan pink salt

¼ cup (30 g) raw cacao nibs, for sprinkling

FOR THE BAR BASE

1 cup (96 g) blanched almond flour

¼ cup (25 g) raw cacao powder

¼ cup (52 g) coconut oil

2 tablespoons maple or coconut syrup

Coconut flakes, freeze dried raspberry, chocolate squares or coins, for garnish

MAKE THE CHOCOLATE-HAZELNUT BUTTER In a medium bowl, combine the h with enough filtered water to cover, add the salt, and soak overnight.

Drain and rinse the soaked hazelnuts with fresh filtered water then drain again and place in a high-speed blender or food processor. Purée on medium-high speed until smooth, about 2 minutes. Add the cacao powder, coconut oil, and honey, pulse a few times, and then purée on medium-high speed until creamy. Add warm water by the tablespoon, as needed, while blending to smooth out the texture. The butter should be smooth and silky with a texture similar to Nutella. After using for the recipe, store the chocolate-hazelnut butter in a glass container in the refrigerator for up to 2 weeks. To bring back to room temperature, leave it out for at least an hour or place the jar in a bowl of warm water.

MAKE THE FUDGE LAYER In a large bowl, combine the cashews and hazelnuts with enough filtered water to cover and a pinch of salt and soak overnight.

Drain and rinse the soaked cashews and hazelnuts with fresh filtered water then drain again and place in a high-speed blender or food processor. Purée on medium-high speed until smooth, about 5 minutes. Add the cacao powder, coconut oil, coconut butter, maple syrup, vanilla powder, and salt and pulse a few times then purée on medium-high speed until creamy. Set aside.

MAKE THE BAR BASE Line a 9 x 13-inch (33 x 23 cm) rectangular pan with unbleached parchment paper with an overhang.

In a large bowl, combine the almond flour, cacao powder, coconut oil, and maple syrup and mix until a dough forms. Press the dough evenly into the parchment-lined pan then freeze until firm, about 30 minutes. Remove the pan from the freezer and pour the fudge batter over the base, spreading it evenly with an offset spatula. Sprinkle with the cacao nibs then freeze for at least 6 hours and preferably overnight.

Use the parchment to remove the bars from the pan and generously spread the chocolate-hazelnut butter. For garnish, add coconut flakes freeze-dried raspberry, and chocolate squares or coins.

Cut into slices and serve. Store the bars in an airtight glass container in the freezer for up to 2 months.

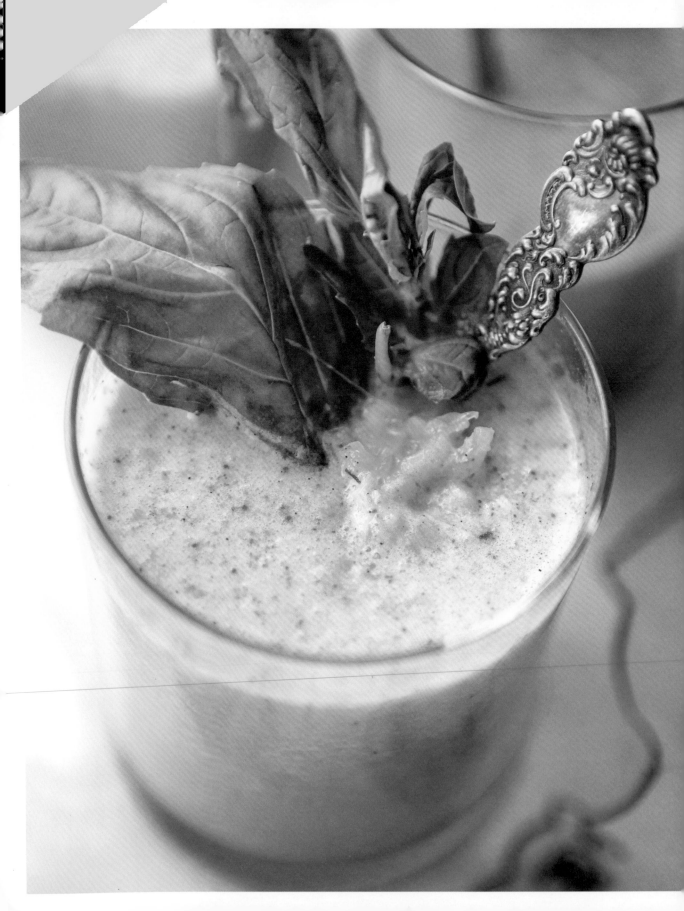

PROBIOTIC VEGAN LASSI

MAKES 1 SERVING

A lassi is not a fancy smoothie, but rather an upgraded version. Unlike a smoothie, in which fruit is the base and main component, the star of a lassi is yogurt or kefir, rich in probiotics and healthy fats. Although traditionally made with dairy yogurt or kefir, a lassi can easily be concocted using dairy-free coconut yogurt. Sweet, slightly tangy coconut yogurt gives a lassi added tropical flair. It's also easier to digest and adds a healthy dose of saturated fats, which help keep you satiated, increase mental agility, and make the nutrients in the fruit more readily available.

You can freeze the banana or mango for a thicker, creamier smoothie, but according to Ayurvedic and Chinese medicine, keeping them at room temperature allows for better digestion and assimilation. Blended foods are already "cooling" or slowing for the digestive system, so further cooling them makes them harder to process.

1 cup (245 g) coconut yogurt (page 179)

1 small ripe banana, chopped or ½ cup (82 g) chopped fresh mango

1 teaspoon ground turmeric

1 teaspoon ground ginger

2 tablespoons fresh lemon juice

Fresh basil, for garnish (optional)

In a high-speed blender, combine the coconut yogurt, banana, turmeric, ginger, and lemon juice and blend until smooth. Serve immediately garnished with fresh basil, if using.

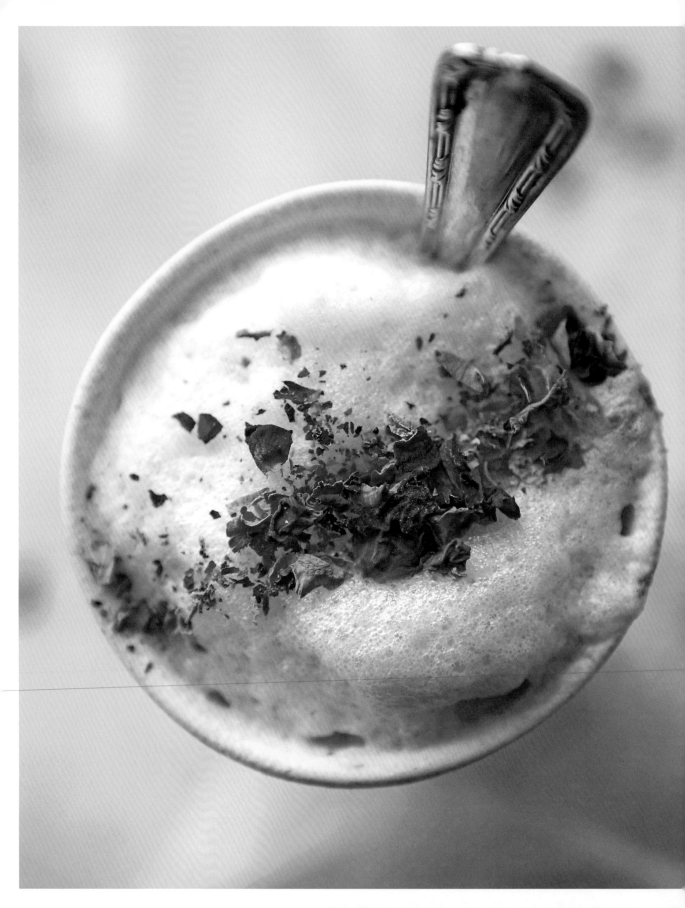

MORNING MORINGA ROSE LATTE

MAKES 1 SERVING

This herbal latte was one of the very first recipes I created following my introduction to adaptogenic herbs. I fell in love with moringa when I discovered it gave me a light buzz of energy without the drawbacks of caffeine. But this miracle leaf does so much more: It's packed with bio-available minerals and high levels of vitamins, such as B12, C, D, and E, making it a food used worldwide to combat malnutrition. It also contains all the essential amino acids, as well as phenolics, including quercetin and kaempferol, which are potent antioxidants that stabilize blood sugar levels, detox and protect the liver, and promote healthy lipid levels.

Rose proves to be the perfect accompaniment with moringa. In Ayurvedic medicine, moringa aids physical digestion by increasing *agni*, or digestive fire, while rose stimulates our emotional digestion, or *sadhak agni*. Although rose is cooling, in an Ayurvedic sense, it enhances *agni* or the digestive fire just as moringa does. This unique quality makes it balancing for all three of the doshas or physical constitutions outlined in Ayurvedic medicine, manifested atop the pillows of this foamy green beverage.

I also added pine pollen, an adaptogenic tonic that's a rich source of minerals and vitamins A, B, D, and E, as well as copper, calcium, and folic acid. Pine pollen also assists in whole-body function, stabilizing hormones, regulating weight by supporting metabolism, detoxifying the liver, and promoting endurance and longevity. Plus, it contains more than twenty amino acids and all eight essential amino acids, making it a nourishing complete protein. Even better.

Lastly, I included lucuma, a creamy, low-glycemic sweetener derived from the lucuma fruit and available in powdered form. By providing a significant dose of fiber and minerals for musculoskeletal regeneration, lucuma soothes tissues and muscle fibers and tames inflammation.

1½ cups (360 ml) hemp milk or milk of your choice

1 tablespoon crushed dried organic rose petals

2 teaspoons coconut oil or ghee

1 teaspoon lucuma powder

1 teaspoon pine pollen

½ teaspoon moringa powder

Pinch of Himalayan pink salt

Stevia (optional)

In a small pot over low heat, gently heat the milk until hot but not boiling.

In a high-speed blender, combine the rose petals, coconut oil, lucuma powder, pine pollen, moringa powder, and salt. Add the warm milk and blend until fully combined. Add the stevia to taste, if using, then blend again and enjoy!

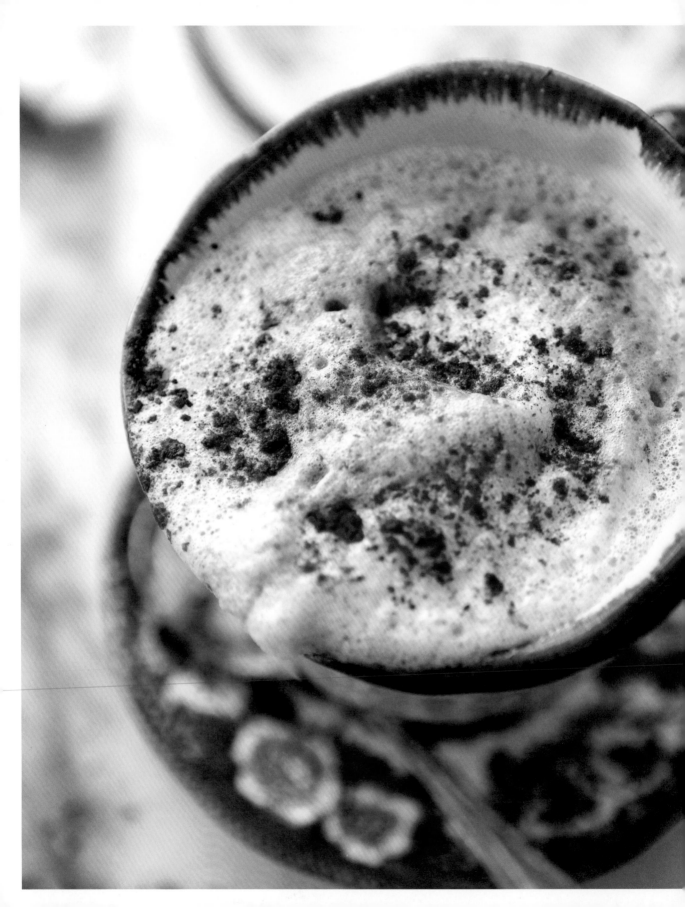

MUSHROOM MAGIC MOCHA

MAKES 1 SERVING

I created this coffee-free mocha to generate some voltage for my morning runs. Cacao-based drinks such as *tejate* have been used throughout history, most famously by the ancient Mayans, as a sacred tonic to boost vitality. It typically combines ingredients like grain and chiles, but the secret is *rosita de cacao*, which provides the drink's froth. This alternative version recreates that with coconut oil instead, obtains its floral notes from rose water, and has the added benefits of mushrooms.

Unlike coffee, which is a stimulant that leads to a crash, cordyceps is an adaptogenic mushroom that stabilizes energy levels. It increases the rate at which ADP (adenosine diphosphate) is converted into ATP (adenosine triphosphate). Cordyceps increases the transportation of these "molecular batteries" by nearly 28 percent![12] It also increases the body's maximum oxygen intake (VO2 max) allowing for increased breathing capacity, benefitting athletes and those suffering from asthma.

Maca powder boosts stamina and prolongs endurance, partially because of its hormone-balancing effect. It stabilizes estrogen and progesterone levels in women, particularly those suffering from the symptoms of menopause or polycystic ovarian syndrome (PCOS). Unlike yellow and red maca, black maca increases testosterone, which is beneficial for sperm production and male reproductive health, and aids in strength and recovery from workouts.

2 tablespoons raw cacao powder

2 teaspoons coconut oil or ghee

2 teaspoons cordyceps powder or 1 packet Four Sigmatic Cordyceps

1 teaspoon maca powder*

¼ teaspoon ground cinnamon

¼ teaspoon ground ginger

¼ teaspoon vanilla powder

⅛ teaspoon rose water (optional)

1 cup (240 ml) water, almond milk, or a plant-based milk of your choice

Stevia (optional)

In a high-speed blender, combine the cacao powder, coconut oil, cordyceps powder, maca powder, cinnamon, ginger, vanilla powder, and rose water, if using. Heat the water or plant-based milk to just below boiling—to avoid damaging the delicate nutrients in the ingredients, avoid boiling the liquid. Carefully add the hot liquid to the blender and purée on high until frothy. Sweeten with stevia to taste, if using.

NOTE *If you have a sensitive stomach, I recommend gelatinized maca powder over the raw version. It takes 9 pounds (4 kg) of raw maca powder to produce 2¼ pounds (1 kg) of the gelatinized version, making it an even more concentrated source of nutrients. However, the heat does alter the enzymes and some nutrients that are preserved in the raw version, including glucosinolates, which are sulfur-containing compounds that are anticancerous and balance thyroid hormones.[13]*

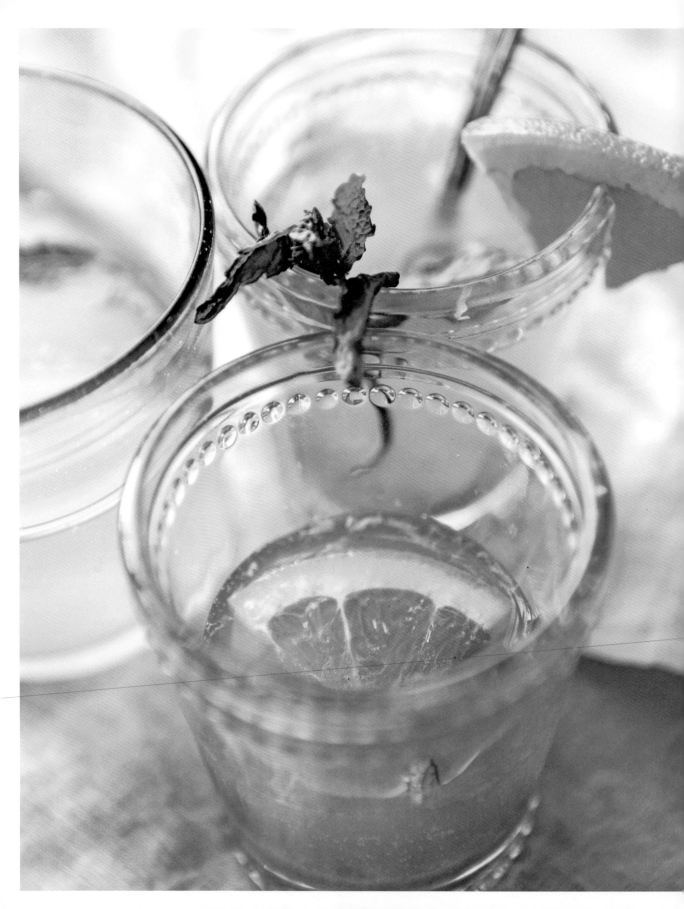

FERMENTED DRINKS

Kombucha is a traditional fermented tea drink that has been brewed and consumed throughout history, and is thought to have been developed in the regions of China, Japan, and Russia.

During the industrial revolution of the eighteenth century, villagers in Russia drank it to fend off the toxic effects of living near factories, while Soviet-era Olympic athletes used it to flush lactic acid from their bodies to prevent sore muscles and build endurance. Kombucha prevents the buildup of natural compounds like lactic acid, as well as environmental toxins, by binding them with organic acids present in the tea and being excreted through the kidneys.[14]

Jun is a lighter sister to kombucha. It's a live, fermented probiotic drink and has the same digestive-enhancing, skin-healing, and mood-boosting properties as kombucha, but with a softer taste and milder effect. Its base is made with green rather than black tea and instead of raw cane sugar it's sweetened with honey. In Ayurvedic medicine, honey is considered one of the ultimate vehicles for delivering the medicinal qualities of herbs, which adds to jun's benefits. Green tea is a source of antioxidants, anti-cancer polyphenols, and L-theanine. Unlike caffeine, L-theanine crosses the blood-brain barrier and induces calm by increasing the activity of the neurotransmitter GABA. It works synergistically with green tea's caffeine to provide a source of calm energy.

To make kombucha and jun you will need scoby. A scoby is the "mother" used to make fermented drinks. It's an acronym that stands for: Symbiotic Culture of Bacteria and Yeast. The scoby is what allows for fermentation and turns the sweet tea base into a tangy, fizzy drink. You can purchase a kombucha scoby from the website Cultures for Health and jun scoby from the website Kombucha Kamp. Or if you know someone who makes their own kombucha, they should be able to provide you with one.

Kombucha

Jun

Kombucha

MAKES 2 QUARTS (ABOUT 2 L)

8 cups (2 l) filtered water

2 teaspoons loose-leaf or 4 bags organic black tea

½ cup (114 g) organic raw cane sugar

1 kombucha scoby plus ½ cup (120 ml) kombucha tea
from an already-cultured batch or store-bought

Chamomile, hibiscus, ginger, fresh fruit,
or the flavoring of your choice (optional)*

Boil the water then remove from the heat, add the tea leaves or bags, and steep for 10 minutes. Remove the tea leaves or bags and pour the tea into a 2-quart or larger glass jar or jug. Add the cane sugar, stir well, and let stand at room temperature until cool to the touch. Add the kombucha scoby and the ½ cup (120 ml) of starter tea. Cover the mouth of the jar with a cheesecloth.

Let the tea ferment at room temperature and away from direct sunlight for at least 1 week and up to 2 weeks. Taste the tea after 1 week and find a ferment time that works for you. I find that 1 week usually isn't enough time for the tea to truly ferment, so I like to let it ferment for about 2 weeks.

Pour the kombucha into glass bottles or jars, reserving ½ cup (120 ml) in the jug to make your next batch. Store the kombucha in the refrigerator for up to 1 week—after that it starts to lose its potency. If you want fizzy kombucha, leave about 3 inches (7.5 cm) of space at the top, seal the container, and let stand at room temperature and away from direct sunlight for 2 to 3 days before refrigerating.

NOTE *To make flavored kombucha, add the herb, root, or fruit of your choice (use 1 tablespoon per 2 cups / 480 ml) to the bottles of finished kombucha and let infuse for 2 to 3 days, while the kombucha is getting fizzy. Adding these flavorings is optional but they do increase fizziness.*

Jun

MAKES 2 QUARTS (ABOUT 2 L)

8 cups (2 l) filtered water
2 teaspoons loose-leaf or 4 bags organic green tea
½ cup (170 g) raw honey
1 jun scoby plus ½ cup (120 ml) jun tea
from an already-cultured batch or store-bought

Boil the water then remove from the heat, add the tea leaves or bags, and steep for 10 minutes.

Remove the tea leaves or bags and pour the tea into a 2-quart or larger glass jar or jug. Let stand at room temperature until cool to the touch. Add the honey and stir until well incorporated. Add the jun scoby and the ½ cup (120 ml) of starter tea. Cover the mouth of the jar with a cheesecloth.

Let the tea ferment at room temperature and away from direct sunlight. Jun is a lighter brew, so it should be ready by the 1 week fermentation mark, depending on your room's temperature. In colder environments, fermentation is slower and will take longer. Adjust the ferment time according to your taste.

Pour the jun into glass bottles or jars, reserving ½ cup (120 ml) in the jug to make your next batch. Store the kombucha in the refrigerator for up to 1 week—after that it starts to lose its potency. If you want fizzy jun, leave about 3 inches (7.5 cm) of space at the top, seal the container, and let stand at room temperature and away from direct sunlight for 2 to 3 days before refrigerating.

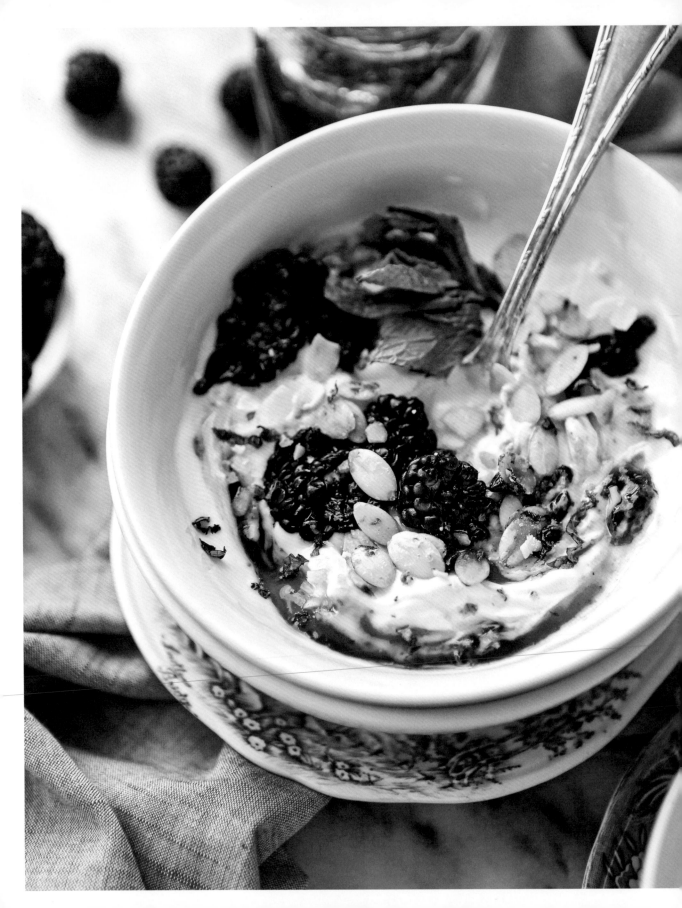

PRESERVING, CULTURING, & FERMENTING

Fermented vegetables are a traditional food in so many cultures and are one of the most potent sources of digestive enzymes. They allow for the proper amount of stomach acid to be released, triggering the production of enzymes to prepare for digestion. In other words, a spoonful of sauerkraut is like nature's version of a before-dinner antacid tablet.

Sauerkraut can also take the place of a probiotic supplement, as the *lactobacilli* bacteria are present not only in higher quantities than are contained in a pill but they are alive. By comparison, almost all the bacteria colonies in most probiotic supplements are weakened by the time, temperature fluctuations, and sometimes over-processing they go through.

The same is true for most store-bought fermented vegetables. Not only are they more expensive and usually contain more brine than vegetables, but some are also partially pasteurized and/or fermented only briefly. You will immediately taste the tangy difference that fermentation time makes with store-bought versus raw, homemade and properly fermented sauerkraut.

For those who have never consumed truly raw or homemade fermented foods, I suggest starting with only a tablespoon before meals. The large amount of probiotics in this sauerkraut can be overwhelming for the body if consumed in high quantities. In proper amounts, sauerkraut protects against pathogens with its probiotics, alkalizes the body; assists in the chelation and removal of heavy metals; promotes nutrient absorption; increases healthy gut flora; and strengthens bones with its calcium, magnesium, and vitamin K content.

Sauerkraut

MAKES 2 QUARTS (ABOUT 2 L)

5 pounds (2.3 kg) green or purple cabbage
4 tablespoons Himalayan pink salt

Before you begin, wash your hands and the cabbages thoroughly. Sanitize a 2-quart (2 L) glass jar with a clamp lid, along with a large bowl, knife, and cutting board. Proper sanitation is critical to ensure that no bacteria contaminate the vessel or the sauerkraut.

Cut each cabbage in half and shred it into thin slices using a knife or in a food processor. I like my sauerkraut chunkier, so I leave the core in and slice the cabbage by hand. Place the shredded cabbage and the salt in the large sanitized bowl and use your hands to massage the cabbage to release its natural juices. Cover the bowl with a clean cloth and let stand for 30 minutes to release more juices.

After 30 minutes, the cabbage should be wilted. Transfer it to the sanitized jar, pressing on the cabbage to compress it and release more juices. There should be about 3 inches (7.5 cm) of space at the top of the jar. If there's more space, add more of the remaining liquid or "brine" from the bowl until there is only 3 inches (7.5 cm) of space at the top. Reserve any remaining brine for later use, such as in salad dressings (page 181).

Clasp the jar shut, clean off any spills or residue, and let ferment, away from direct sunlight and without opening the jar, for 2 months. If your home runs cooler, let ferment for 2½ months. Once opened, store the sauerkraut in the refrigerator for up to 6 months.

NOTE *This recipe produces about 5 pounds (2.3 kg) of sauerkraut for $4, whereas most sauerkraut sells for about $11 for 1 pound (450 g).*

Cultured Coconut Yogurt

MAKES ABOUT 1½ CUPS (340 G)

1 (13.5 ounce/398 ml) can full-fat coconut milk

3 teaspoons probiotic powder or powder from capsules
(enough to provide 15 to 20 billion cfu)

Shake the can of coconut milk to ensure the liquid and cream are well mixed. In a large glass bowl, combine the coconut milk and probiotic powder and stir well. Cover the container with a cheesecloth and place in a dark, cool area for 24 to 48 hours. Taste the yogurt after 24 hours—it should be tangy, which is a cue that it's done. If not, continue to ferment the yogurt for another 24 hours.

Transfer the cheesecloth-covered bowl to the refrigerator and let the yogurt stand for 3 more days to thicken; stir it once a day to keep it smooth. Store the yogurt in glass containers in the refrigerator for up to 1 month.

Preserved Lemons

MAKES ABOUT 2 QUARTS (2 L)

2 pounds (900 g) soft, juicy lemons

¼ cup (72 g) Himalayan pink salt

Wash the lemons and carefully cut off the ends. Cut the lemons in half. Cut the lemon halves into quarters, cutting only about ⅔ of the way through, so that the base remains intact. Rub the salt inside and all over the lemons then place them in a sanitized glass container, jar, or fermentation crock. Sprinkle any remaining salt over the lemons and muddle them with the back of a spoon until they soften and release enough juice to be completely coated. Seal the jar and let the lemons ferment at room temperature and away from direct sunlight or heat—in a dark cupboard—for 1 month. Store the preserved lemons in the refrigerator for up to 2 years.

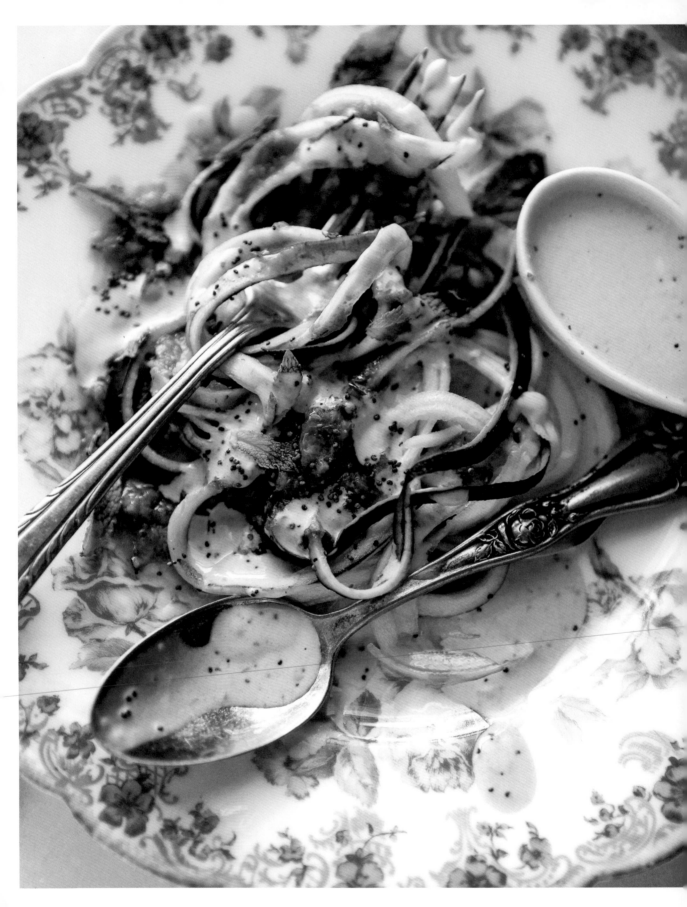

CULTURED DRESSINGS

Fermented salad dressings are the most convenient way to add functional enzymes and probiotics to meals, while also avoiding the unsavory ingredients found in store-bought versions. Most commercially made dressings contain unpronounceable or inflammatory, allergenic ingredients, such as dairy, processed vegetable oils, and hidden sugars. Some even contain neurotoxic monosodium glutamate (MSG), concealed in the form of hydrolyzed vegetable protein or "natural flavor." Additional preservatives, stabilizers, artificial flavors or colors, and oils that are processed at high temperatures and often rancid add further insult to injury.

But while commercial options can lead to digestive upset, inflammation, and disease, the fermented ingredients in these cultured dressings tame inflammation, boost healthy gut flora via probiotics, and counter any toxins that are stored in fat cells by flushing the cells with the healthy fats they each contain.

Mint Medley Dressing

MAKES ABOUT 1½ CUPS (350 ML)

¼ cup (60 ml) freshly squeezed lemon juice

¼ cup (60 ml) freshly squeezed orange juice

¼ cup (60 ml) brine from fermented vegetables, such as sauerkraut (page 178)

4 cloves garlic, peeled

½ cup fresh mint leaves

½ cup (120 ml) extra-virgin olive oil

¼ teaspoon Himalayan pink salt

⅛ teaspoon black pepper

In a high-speed blender, combine the lemon and orange juice, brine, garlic, and mint and purée. With the blender running, slowly add the olive oil and continue blending until thoroughly emulsified. Add the salt and pepper and adjust seasonings to taste. Use the dressing immediately or store in an airtight glass container in the refrigerator for up to 2 weeks.

Preserved Lemon–Poppy Seed Dressing

MAKES ABOUT 1½ CUPS (350 ML)

1 preserved lemon, cut up (page 179)

¼ cup (60 ml) freshly squeezed lemon juice

¼ cup (85g) raw or Manuka honey

2 cloves garlic, peeled

½ tablespoon poppy seeds

1 teaspoon brown mustard*

⅔ cup (150 ml) extra-virgin olive oil

¼ teaspoon Himalayan pink salt

⅛ teaspoon black pepper

In a high-speed blender, combine the preserved lemon, lemon juice, honey, garlic, poppy seeds, and brown mustard and purée. With the blender running, slowly add the olive oil and continue blending until thoroughly emulsified. Add the salt and pepper and adjust seasonings to taste. Use the dressing immediately or store in an airtight glass container in the refrigerator for up to 2 weeks.

NOTE   *Make sure your mustard doesn't contain artificial flavors, vegetable oils, sugar, or distilled, grain-based vinegars. I prefer Eden Food's organic brown mustard, which is stone-ground with apple cider vinegar, another probiotic-rich fermented ingredient.*

Turmeric-Kombucha Vinaigrette

MAKES ABOUT 1 CUP (230 ML) ·

⅓ cup (75 ml) plain kombucha (page 174)

1 tablespoon brown mustard

1 tablespoon raw or Manuka honey (optional)

½ teaspoon ground turmeric

½ teaspoon garlic powder*

⅓ cup (75 ml) extra-virgin olive oil

¼ teaspoon Himalayan pink salt

⅛ teaspoon black pepper

In a small bowl, whisk together the kombucha and brown mustard. Add the honey, if using, along with the turmeric and garlic powder and whisk again. Slowly add the olive oil, whisking constantly to emulsify the vinaigrette. Add the salt and pepper and adjust seasonings to taste. To create a creamier variation, add a ¼ cup (61 g) cultured coconut yogurt (page 179). Use the vinaigrette immediately or store in an airtight glass container in the refrigerator for up to 2 weeks.

NOTE *Make sure your garlic powder is free from any anti-caking agents, sugar, or additives. I prefer Badia spices, which are also certified gluten-free.*

Tangy Ranch Dressing

MAKES ABOUT 1½ CUPS (350 ML)

1½ cups (375 g) coconut yogurt (page 179)
¼ cup (5 g) minced fresh flat-leaf parsley
2 cloves garlic, minced
1 tablespoon freshly squeezed lemon juice
1 tablespoon onion powder
2 tablespoons olive oil
½ teaspoon Himalayan pink salt

In a high-speed blender, combine the coconut yogurt, parsley, garlic, lemon juice, and onion powder and purée. With the blender running, slowly add the olive oil and continue blending until thoroughly emulsified. Add the salt and adjust seasoning to taste. Use the dressing immediately or store in an airtight glass container in the refrigerator for up to 2 weeks.

NOTES

FARMACY

1 Ballantyne, Sarah, "Gluten Cross-Reactivity: How your body can still think you're eating gluten even after giving it up," The Paleo Mom (blog), February 28, 2017, accessed May 1, 2017, https://www.thepaleomom.com/gluten-cross-reactivity-update-how-your-body-can-still-think-youre-eating-gluten-even-after-giving-it-up/.

2 Tarash, Igal, and Aristo Vojdani, "Cross-Reaction between Gliadin and Different Food and Tissue Antigens," *Food and Nutrition Sciences* 4, no. 1 (2013), accessed May 1, 2017, doi:10.4236/fns.2013.41005.

3 "Magnesium," National Institutes of Health: Office of Dietary Supplements, February 11, 2016, accessed May 1, 2017, https://ods.od.nih.gov/factsheets/Magnesium-HealthProfessional/.

4 Houghton, Lisa A., and Reinhold Vieth, "The case against ergocalciferol (vitamin D2) as a vitamin supplement," The American Journal of Clinical Nutrition, October 01, 2006, accessed June 22, 2017, http://ajcn.nutrition.org/content/84/4/694.full.

5 INTERPHONE Study Group, "Brain tumour risk in relation to mobile telephone use: results of the INTERPHONE international case-control study," *International Journal of Epidemiology* 39, no. 3 (June 2010): 675–94, accessed May 1, 2017. doi: 10.1093/ije/dyq079.

6 Adams, Jessica A., Sandro C. Esteves, Tamara S. Galloway, Fiona Mathews, and Debapriya Mondal, "Effect of mobile telephones on sperm quality: a systematic review and meta-analysis," *Environment International* 70 (September 2014): 106–112, accessed May 1, 2017, doi:10.1016/j.envint.2014.04.015.

7 Brown, S.S., J.A.H. Forrest, and P. Roscoe, "A Controlled Trial Of Fructose In The Treatment Of Acute Alcoholic Intoxication," *The Lancet* 300, no. 7783 (October 28, 1972): 898–900, doi:10.1016/s0140-6736(72)92533-0.

8 Sprince, Herbert, Clarence M. Parker, George G. Smith, and Leon J. Gonzales, "Protection against Acetaldehyde Toxicity in the rat byl-cysteine, thiamin andl-2-Methylthiazolidine-4-carboxylic acid," *Agents and Actions* 4, no. 2 (April 4, 1974): 125–30, doi:10.1007/bf01966822.

9 "Some Pain Drugs Increase the Risk of Heart Attack," *Mayo Clinic*, April 26, 2013, accessed May 01, 2017, http://newsnetwork.mayoclinic.org/discussion/some-pain-drugs-increase-the-risk-of-heart-attack/.

10 Asakura, Hiroyuki, Tatsuya Hayashi, and Tamaki Matsumoto, "Does lavender aromatherapy alleviate premenstrual emotional symptoms?: a randomized crossover trial," *Biopsychosocial Medicine* 3, no. 2 (2013), accessed May 1, 2017, doi:10.1186/1751-0759-7-12.

11 Hsu, Tsung-Fu, Andrew C. Lai, Chia-Ching Lin, Yu-Ting Lin, and Ming-Chiu Ou, "Pain relief assessment by aromatic essential oil massage on outpatients with primary dysmenorrhea: a randomized, double-blind clinical trial," *Journal of Obstetrics and Gynaecology Research* 38, no. 5 (May 2012): 817–22, accessed May 1, 2017, doi:10.1111/j.1447-0756.2011.01802.x.

12 *Behind the Dazzling Smile*, Cornucopia Institute (July 2016): 2–3, https://www.cornucopia.org/wp-content/uploads/2016/08/toothpaste-report-web.pdf.

13 Farajzadeh, Matthew, Chenyuan Pan, Wenhui Qiu, Nancy L. Wayne, Ming Yang, and Yali Zhao, "Actions of Bisphenol A and Bisphenol S on the Reproductive Neuroendocrine System During Early Development in Zebrafish," *Endocrinology* 157, no. 2 (February 2016): 636–47, accessed May 1, 2017, doi:10.1210/en.2015-1785.

SPIRITUAL SMACK

1   Ellyard, Lawrence, *Reiki Healer: A Complete Guide to the Path and Practice of Reiki* (Twin Lakes, WI: Lotus Press, 2004).

2   Wallace, David Foster. *This is Water: Some Thoughts, Delivered on a Significant Occasion, about Living a Compassionate Life* (Boston: Little, Brown and Company, 2009).

BEAUTY BITES

1   Benbrook CM, Butler G, Latif MA, Leifert C, Davis DR, "Organic production enhances milk nutritional quality by shifting fatty acid composition: A United States–wide, 18-month study," *PLOS ONE* 8, no. 12, https://doi.org/10.1371/journal.pone.0082429.

2   Favell, D.J., "A Comparison of the vitamin C content of fresh and frozen vegetables," *Food Chemistry* 62, no. 1 (1998): 5p-64, http://ucanr.edu/datastoreFiles/608-97.pdf.

3   Barrett, Diane M., Christine M. Bruhn, and Joy C. Rickman, "Nutritional comparison of fresh, frozen and canned fruits and vegetables. Part 1. Vitamins C and B and phenolic compounds," *Journal of the Science of Food and Agriculture* 87 (2007): 930–44, http://ucce.ucdavis.edu/files/datastore/234-779.pdf.

4   Rubin, Beverly S., "Bisphenol A: An endocrine disruptor with widespread exposure and multiple effects," *The Journal of Steroid Biochemistry and Molecular Biology* 127, no. 1–2 (October 2011): 27–34, doi:https://doi.org/10.1016/j.jsbmb.2011.05.002.

5   Abbott, et al., "A review of fatty acid," *Nutrition Journal* 9, no. 10 (2010).

6   Abbott, Amber, Cynthia A. Daley, Patrick S. Doyle, Stephanie Larson, and Glenn A. Nadar, "A review of fatty acid profiles and antioxidant content in grass-fed and grain-fed beef," *Nutrition Journal* 9, no. 10 (2010), http://doi.org/10.1186/1475-2891-9-10.

7   Boyce, J., J.C. Brooks, E. Hentges, L. Hoover, J.C. Howe, J.M. Leheska, M.F. Miller, B. Shriver, and L.D. Thompson, "Effects of conventional and grass-feeding systems on the nutrient composition of beef," *Journal of Animal Science* 86 (2008): 3575–85. doi:10.2527/jas.2007-0565.

8   Amaro-Lopez, M., R. Moreno-Rojas, and G. Zurera-Cosano, "Effect of processing on contents and relationships of mineral elements of milk," *Food Chemistry* 51, no. 1 (1994): 75–8, https://doi.org/10.1016/0308-8146(94)90050-7.

9   Barański, Marcin, Dominika Średnicka-Tober, Nikolaos Volakakis, Chris Seal, Roy Sanderson, Gavin B. Stewart, Charles Benbrook, et. al., "Higher antioxidant and lower cadmium concentrations and lower incidence of pesticide residues in organically grown crops: a systematic literature review and meta-analyses," *British Journal of Nutrition* 112, no. 5 (2014): 794–811. doi:10.1017/S0007114514001366.

10 Joseph, Thangam, David Joy, R. Rajendran, Guido Shoba, and R.S.S.R. Srinivas, "Influence of piperine on the pharmacokinetics of curcumin in animals and human volunteers," *Planta Medica* 64, no. 4 (January 2007): 353–56, doi:10.1055/s-2006-957450.

11 Johnson, I.T., "Glucosinolates: Bioavailability and importance to health," *International Journal for Vitamin and Nutrition Research* 72 (2002): 26–31, doi:https://doi.org/10.1024/0300-9831.72.1.26.

12 Rogers, Robert, *The Fungal Pharmacy: The Complete Guide to Medicinal Mushrooms and Lichens of North America* (Berkeley: North Atlantic Books, 2011).

13 Johnson, Ian. T., "Glucosinolates," *International Journal for Vitamin and Nutrition Research* 72 (January 2002), 26–31.

14 Reid, G., J. Jass, M. T. Sebulsky, and J. K. McCormick, "Potential uses of probiotics in clinical practice," *Clinical Microbiology Reviews* (October 2003), accessed June 20, 2017, https://www.ncbi.nlm.nih.gov/pubmed/14557292.

ACKNOWLEDGMENTS

I would first like to thank my editor, **Holly La Due**, for seeing and believing in my work, allowing me to further believe in myself. She has given me more gifts than just this book to behold. I'm also grateful for **Laura Palese**, our designer, and to **Sophie Golub**, **Luke Chase**, and the rest of the **Prestel team** who assisted in the realization of this book.

I would like to thank **Hanna Rhodes**, my best friend turned assistant photographer. I am thankful also to the **Marlton Hotel** in New York for providing space to capture some of these photos.

Also, I am thankful for my **family and friends** who have encouraged me along the way. **My sister**, **my uncle**, and **my aunt** foremost. Last but not least: I would like to express my gratitude for **all those who have supported me** whose names I keep privately in my heart.

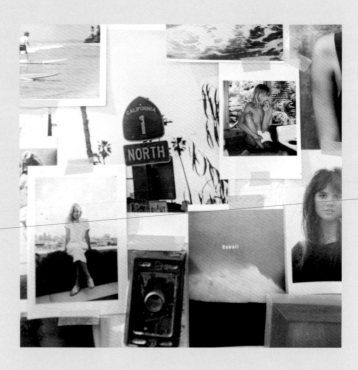

INDEX